# 60 tips

# detox

Marie Borrel

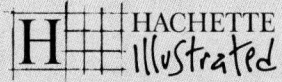

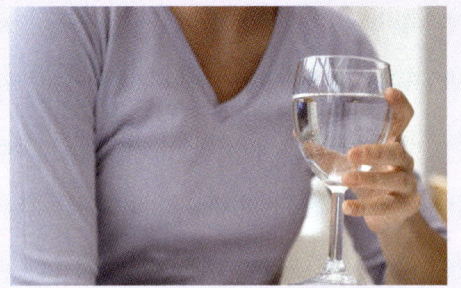
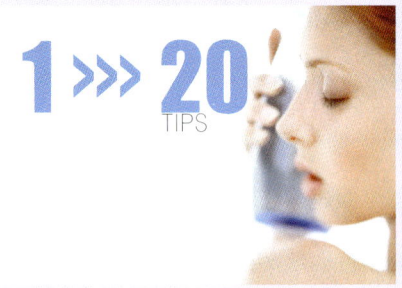

# contents

introduction 4
how to use this book 7
does your body really need a detox? 8

useful addresses 124
index 125
acknowledgements 126

Note: The information and recommendations given in this book are not intended to be a substitute for medical advice. Consult your doctor before acting on any recommendations given in this book. The authors and publisher disclaim any liability, loss, injury or damage incurred as a consequence, directly or indirectly, of the use and application of the contents of this book.

# 1 >>> 20 TIPS

| 01 | drink water, then more water | 12 |
| 02 | eat organic | 14 |
| 03 | cut out sugars and animal fats | 16 |
| 04 | make good use of aromatic herbs | 18 |
| 05 | you must give up smoking! | 20 |
| 06 | cut down on coffee and alcohol | 22 |
| 07 | give up animal products | 24 |
| 08 | eat more raw food | 26 |
| 09 | in springtime try a strawberry diet | 28 |
| 10 | in summer try a cherry diet | 30 |
| 11 | in autumn try a grape diet | 31 |
| 12 | fasting? – take great care | 32 |
| 13 | fruit and veg are good for the liver | 34 |
| 14 | fruit and veg are good for the kidneys | 36 |
| 15 | fruit and veg for healthy bowels | 38 |
| 16 | try a course of lemon juice | 40 |
| 17 | drink clay | 41 |
| 18 | eat plenty of fibre | 42 |
| 19 | drink tea, then more tea | 44 |
| 20 | don't confuse detox with slimming | 46 |
|  | case study | 47 |

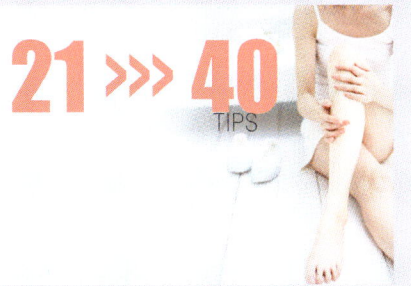 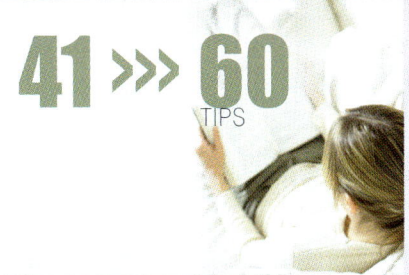

# 21 »> 40 TIPS

| | | |
|---|---|---|
| 21 | sweat it out | 50 |
| 22 | get moving! | 52 |
| 23 | herbal teas to make you sweat | 54 |
| 24 | plants that are good for the skin | 56 |
| 25 | treat yourself to lymphatic drainage | 58 |
| 26 | massage your feet | 60 |
| 27 | plants that are good for the kidneys | 62 |
| 28 | poultices will do the trick | 64 |
| 29 | eat plenty of charcoal | 66 |
| 30 | buy a hot-water bottle | 67 |
| 31 | the olive: a tree of many talents | 68 |
| 32 | plants that are good for the liver | 70 |
| 33 | beating constipation | 72 |
| 34 | plants that are good for the intestines | 74 |
| 35 | consider colonic irrigation | 76 |
| 36 | have a really good laugh | 77 |
| 37 | massage your stomach | 78 |
| 38 | take a deep breath | 80 |
| 39 | plants that are good for breathing | 82 |
| 40 | take your time | 84 |
| | case study | 85 |

# 41 »> 60 TIPS

| | | |
|---|---|---|
| 41 | come to terms with stress | 88 |
| 42 | learn to relax | 90 |
| 43 | little bottles of floral essence | 92 |
| 44 | elixirs to quell your fears | 94 |
| 45 | elixirs to boost morale | 95 |
| 46 | try homeopathy | 96 |
| 47 | a bath fit for a goddess! | 98 |
| 48 | let massage help you | 100 |
| 49 | upside-down breathing | 102 |
| 50 | close your eyes and visualize | 104 |
| 51 | massage your solar plexus | 105 |
| 52 | don't skimp on magnesium | 106 |
| 53 | drive away negative thoughts | 108 |
| 54 | express yourself! | 110 |
| 55 | make them take 'no' for an answer | 112 |
| 56 | stop feeling guilty | 114 |
| 57 | drive out the green-eyed monster | 116 |
| 58 | make a date with nature | 118 |
| 59 | take a seaside holiday | 120 |
| 60 | enjoy it! | 122 |
| | case study | 123 |

# introduction

## Cleansing body and mind

For thousands of years, people have known that the human body should be 'cleansed' at least once a year in order to stay healthy. All the major religions have purification rites: for instance, Christianity has Lent, Islam Ramadan, and Hinduism Durga Puja. This is no coincidence. These are strategies that help to address the fact that our bodies become 'polluted', just like the inner workings of a gas boiler or a car engine. When this happens, slowly but insidiously, we grow tired, feel anxious, and start to suffer from insomnia. Our minds fare no better, as they become 'polluted' with the stresses and burdens of modern life. We need to put a stop to this and take better care of ourselves.

## Toxins both inside and out

Metabolic processes are taking place continually inside us, and the waste matter from these processes is clogging us up. Each day, in every one of us, several billion cells die, and the body must dispose of all of them. Then there is the food we eat, which is a source of toxins, as well as nutrients, even when it's of the highest quality. In order to be utilized by the body, all food has to be broken down by the digestive system, and this produces waste. For example, before the body is able to recycle them, proteins must be broken down into amino acids, which produce uric acid.

In addition to the food itself, though, we have to deal with more well-known toxins. Besides the bacteria and fungi that might make us seriously ill, we swallow an enormous number of other pollutants that accumulate inside our bodies. We inhale harmful gases, eat chemical colouring agents and additives and take courses of drugs that may have damaging side-effects.

## The excretory organs are not always up to the task

Our body is equipped with several organs – the liver, the kidneys, the lungs and the skin – which contribute to the excretion of waste matter. Sometimes, however, they have too much to do and cannot cope. Then the waste accumulates, just as rubbish does during a dustmen's strike. Our cells are deprived of nourishment, our bodily functions slow down and our whole body begins to find it hard going. If we're not careful, we fall ill. Stress may then exacerbate the problem. When our brain and nervous system are overworked, they take some of the key nutrients that the excretory organs require to eliminate waste. To make matters worse, as we become more tense, we consume more stimulants – such as coffee, alcohol and tea – and we tend to eat less healthily. It's a vicious circle!

## Our helpless body cells!

All our bodily tissues, including the organs, comprise billions of cells. Each cell is a micro-organism that is fed, performs its functions, dies and then is removed as waste. While active, it must be supplied with oxygen and nutrients to act as catalyst and fuel, and needs to be linked to a system which removes its waste products. These vital functions are carried out by bodily fluids, mainly the lymph and interstitial fluids (those between the cells).

If all our body's cells were spread out on the ground, they would cover about 200 hectares and be irrigated by a network of capillaries 10,000km long! On average, the blood takes a minute to complete a circuit of the body, delivering nutrients and removing waste: it's an arduous task. If the excretory organs do not filter out the waste from your blood and remove it from the body, your system will grow sluggish and the whole body may begin to suffer.

As a result of this sluggishness, the body's cells may well be undernourished, not because there is a shortage of oxygen and nutrients, but because the supply system is inefficient. Vitamin and mineral supplements may help, but they cannot solve the problem entirely, as the accumulation of waste will still prevent full nourishment of the cells.

Fortunately, there are simple, natural solutions: avoiding certain foods, fasting for a short time, monodiets, herbal treatments and cleansing the lymphatic system. These should be used in conjunction with relaxation and stress-relief techniques to purify the whole being, body and soul!

# how to use this book

This book offers a made-to-measure programme, which will enable you to deal with your own particular problem. It is organized into four sections:

- **A questionnaire** to help you to assess the extent of your problem.
- **The first 20 tips** that will show you how to change your daily life in order to prevent problems and maintain health and fitness.
- **20 slightly more radical tips** that will develop the subject and enable you to cope when problems occur.
- **The final 20 tips** which are intended for more serious cases, when preventative measures and attempted solutions have not worked.

At the end of each section someone with the same problem as you shares his or her experiences.

You can go methodically through the book from tip I to 60 putting each piece of advice into practice. Alternatively, you can pick out the recommendations which appear to be best suited to your particular case, or those which fit most easily into your daily routine. Or, finally, you can choose to follow the instructions according to whether you wish to prevent problems occurring or cure ones that already exist.

---

> FOR YOUR GUIDANCE

> A symbol at the bottom of each page will help you to identify the natural solutions available:

 **Herbal medicine, aromatherapy, homeopathy, Dr Bach's flower remedies** – how natural medicine can help.

 **Simple exercises** – preventing problems by strengthening your body.

 **Massage and manipulation** – how they help to promote well-being.

 **Healthy eating** – all you need to know about the contribution it makes.

 **Practical tips for** your daily life – so that you can prevent instead of having to cure.

 **Psychology, relaxation, Zen** – advice to help you be at peace with yourself and regain serenity.

> A complete programme that will solve all your health problems.
> Try it!

# Does your body really need a detox?

How many of the statements below apply to you? Answer honestly!

| | | | | | |
|---|---|---|---|---|---|
| yes | no | 1 I eat a lot of meat. | yes | no | 7 I smoke regularly. |
| yes | no | 2 I am always tense and stressed | yes | no | 8 I never say what I think and feel. |
| yes | no | 3 I don't like fruit or vegetables. | yes | no | 9 I never take vitamin or mineral supplements. |
| yes | no | 4 I'm often constipated. | | | |
| yes | no | 5 I suffer from colds and flu every winter. | | | |
| yes | no | 6 I often get spots. | | | |

If statements 1, 2 and 7 apply to you, Tips **1** to **20** are most relevant to you.

If statements 4, 5 and 6 apply to you, turn directly to Tips **21** to **40**.

If statements 2, 8 and 9 apply to you, make Tips **41** to **60** your priority.

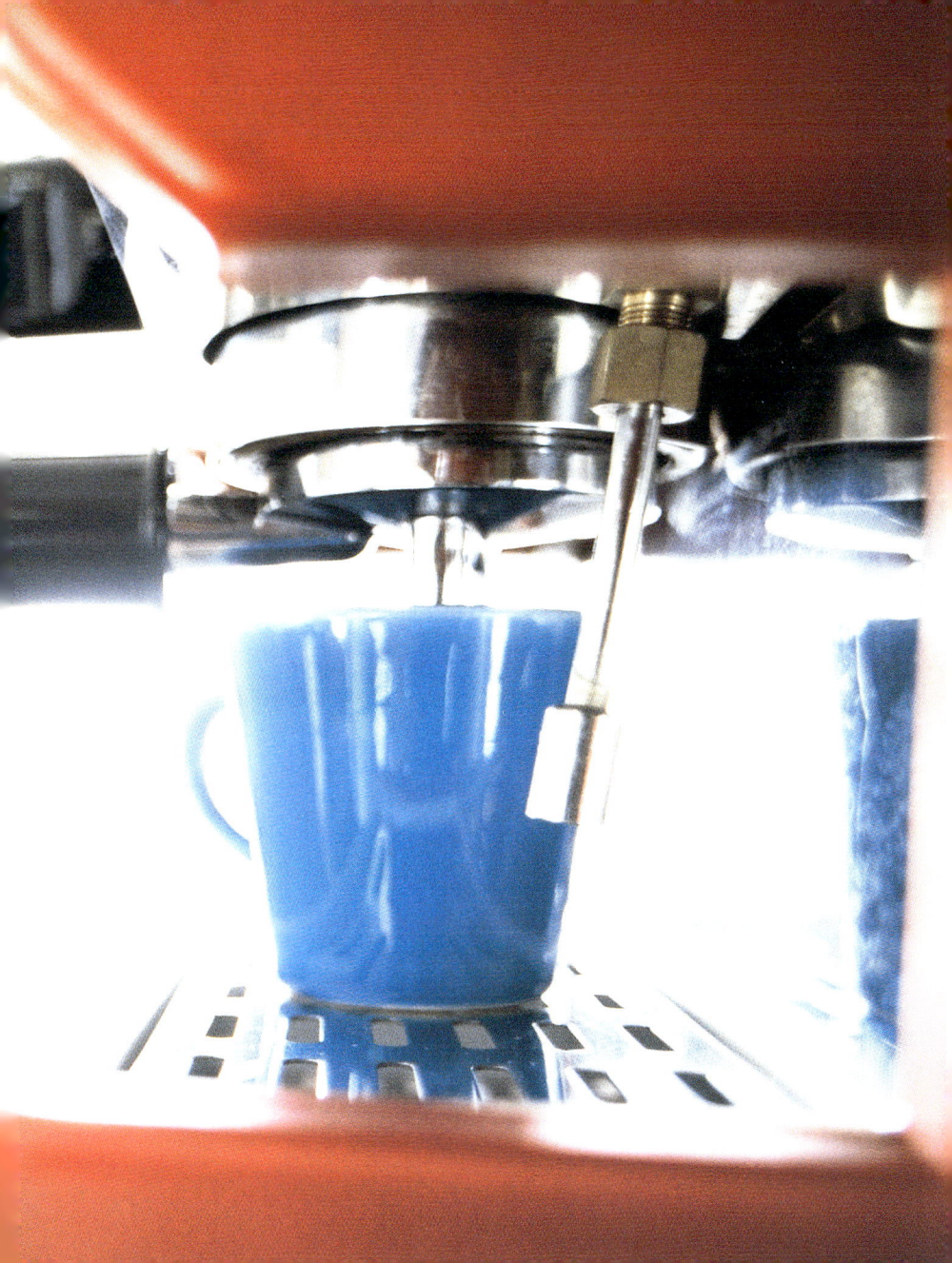

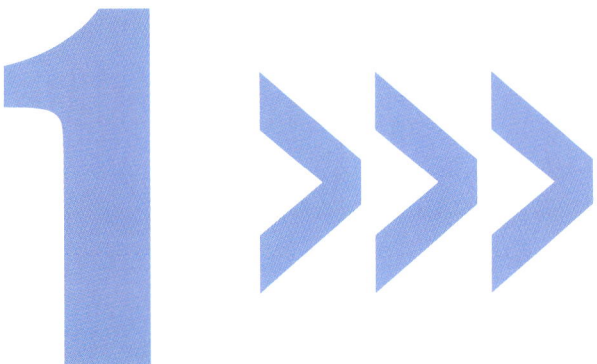

》 Toxins usually accumulate in our bodies because of our diet: we eat too much, our food intake is unbalanced and too often produced in factories. **Changing what we eat is the first step towards cleansing our bodies.**

》》》 But this doesn't mean that we have to eat much less, **just more sensibly.** We need to cut down on food that produces many toxins in favour of food that helps us to dispose of waste matter.

》》》》》 **Eating more fresh vegetables** or trying a monodiet is a good way to start your detox programme.

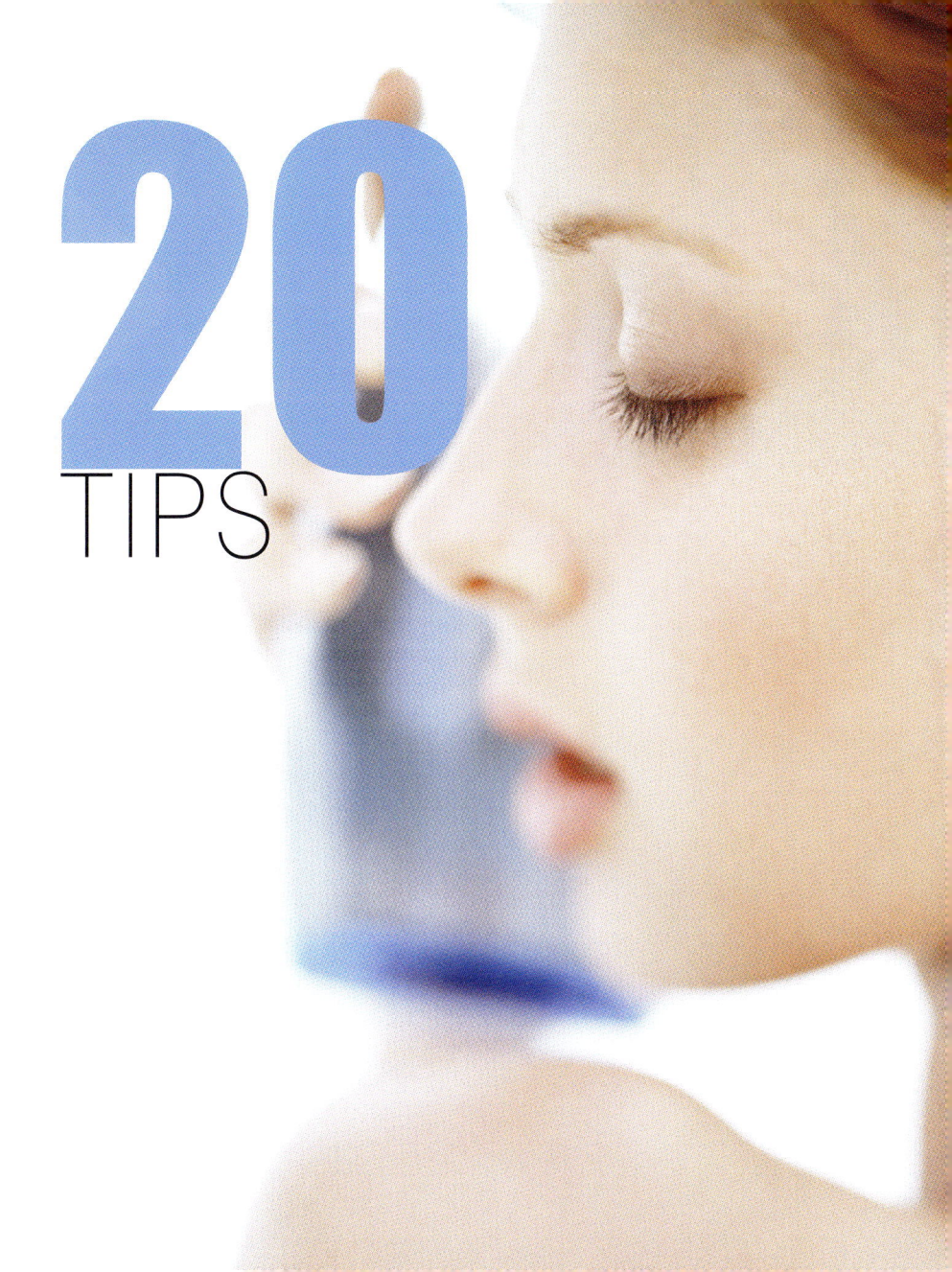

# 20
## TIPS

## 01 drink water, then more water

We need water to wash the outside of our bodies: we wouldn't feel clean without a good shower or bath. But water is also vital for washing us on the inside. Without it, the excretory system cannot function. So, get drinking!

### The solvent that keeps us alive

Water is a solvent that dissolves many substances and transports them around the body. It carries both the nutrients our body needs to function and the waste produced by cellular metabolism. The ceaseless circulation of water inside us is regulated by a complex process involving neurotransmitters (hormones produced by the brain), minerals and the organs concerned with filtration and

● ● ● DID YOU KNOW?

> When a baby is in the womb, it receives water from its mother. Dr Batmanghelidj, a specialist in problems caused by dehydration, believes that morning sickness, often experienced during the early months of pregnancy, could be due to lack of water.

> To ensure the cells, and therefore all the body's functions, are working effectively, an adult needs a regular and adequate supply of water. Without it, the body becomes chronically dehydrated (a condition that is easily overlooked) and vulnerable to illness.

excretion. This system must be working smoothly if the body is to dispose of its waste products and toxins quickly.

## Drink before you get thirsty

To ensure that excretion takes place efficiently, you need to drink! Above all, drink before you are thirsty, because the sensation of thirst indicates that the body is already short of water and so is unable to carry out all its functions, including excretion.

And don't think that any liquid will do. Only water fits the bill. Although herbal teas are useful in cleaning out the body (see Tip 23), they can't replace water. As a general rule, you should drink around 1.5 litres (2½ pints) of water daily, and try to find one that does not have too high a mineral content.

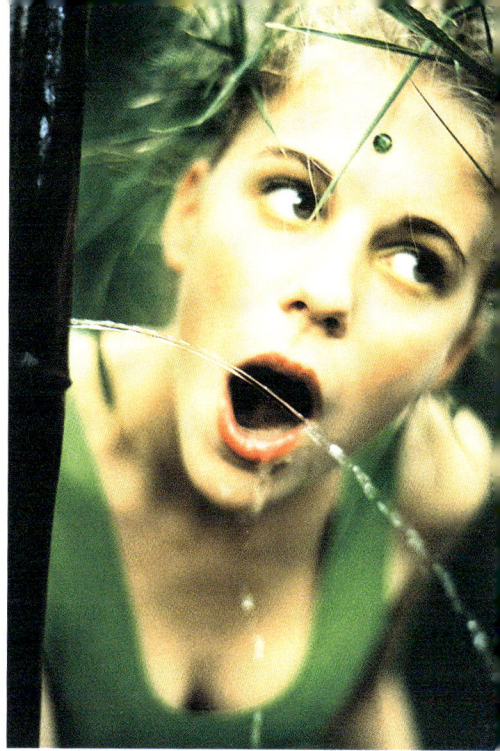

> This problem is particularly acute among elderly people, because they often lose the sensation of thirst.

KEY FACTS

* You absolutely must drink water to cleanse the body and remove toxins.

* Nothing can take the place of water. The best water has a low mineral content.

* The average person needs a litre and a half a day.

## 02 eat organic

Modern food is 'polluted' by substances that contribute to the number of toxins in the body: the residues of chemicals used during the growing of crops or the rearing of animals; additives and colouring agents used in the mass production of food. To avoid these substances, eat organic food.

### Both fresh food and processed food are affected

In industrialized countries it is virtually impossible to live entirely on home-grown food. We have no option but to consume products supplied by the food industry. With fresh food – such as fruit, vegetables and meat – pesticides, chemical fertilizers and antibiotics may all be

● ● ● DID YOU KNOW?

> Organic products are not just chemical-free. Several common procedures cannot be used on any foodstuff that is labelled 'organic'. Irradiation (exposing food to gamma rays to extend its shelf life) is an example of this.

> No one knows whether this process, which modifies the molecular structure of the food, is harmful or not. But it's best to avoid irradiated food if you want to detox your body. Genetically modified products similarly cannot be labelled 'organic'.

present. With processed food – such as bread, pasta, tinned and vacuum-packed products, and fizzy drinks – preservatives, colours, sweeteners and other additives are usually included in the lists of ingredients.

Of course, we mustn't blame these substances for everything. However, they do add to the amount of toxins in the body, and you should avoid them if you want your detox programme to work.

## Look out for the word 'Organic' on the label

The simplest way to ensure you're eating nothing but healthy foods is to go organic. Foodstuffs produced by non-intensive farming methods are subject to very thorough inspections and must satisfy extremely strict requirements. For example, fruit and vegetables must be grown without the use of chemicals and at a specified minimum distance from main roads. Meat must come from animals reared without antibiotics and that are fed only on natural, chemical-free products.

To plot a path through the jungle of food on sale, always check the label.

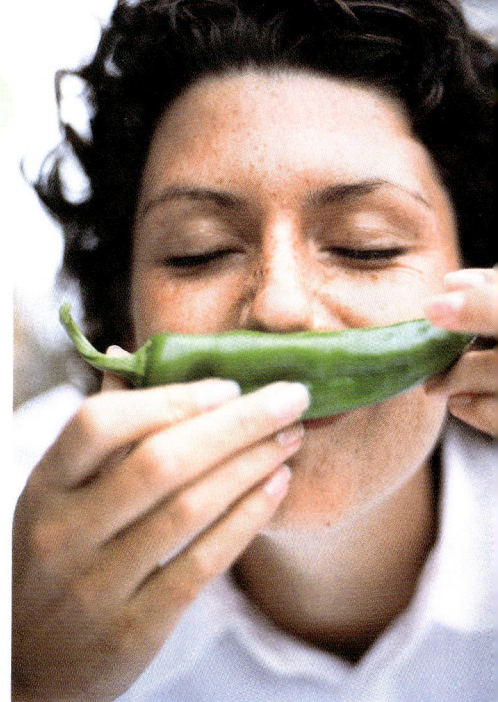

### KEY FACTS

∗ To cleanse the body, you need to eat as healthily and as naturally as you can.

∗ Eat organic food if you are detoxing.

∗ Get into the habit of always checking the label.

## 03
## cut out sugars and animal fats

Before eating a lot of fruit and vegetables, or embarking on a monodiet, ease yourself into your detox programme by avoiding foods that pollute your body and do it no good. Animal fats and refined sugars should be the first items to go.

### No more butter, cheese, sweets and fizzy drinks!

The time has come to choose the food you'll eat during your detox programme. First, give your body some respite by cutting down on animal fats and refined sugars. This is a valuable habit to adopt, because these substances do you no good. Animal fats (butter, cream, cheese and so on), especially when cooked, increase the cholesterol level in the

### ● ● ● DID YOU KNOW?

> Don't worry about the possibility of suffering from a lack of sugar. Even if you never eat these products, your body will still be able to get all the energy it needs from fructose in fruit and, above all, from slow-release sugars in cereals and legume (pod) vegetables. It can also break down fat for energy.

> As for fats themselves, your body will benefit if you eat good essential fatty acids and avoid bad ones. The good ones are found in abundance in vegetable oils and oily fish. The bad ones are in animal fats.

blood and thicken the artery walls. Ketones, toxic compounds, are produced when fat is metabolized. These need to be expelled for the body to remain healthy, so the fewer of them in the bloodstream, the better.

Refined sugars (white sugar, fizzy drinks, sweets, jams and so on) are rapidly absorbed from the gut and so cause a rush of glucose into the blood. This high concentration of glucose in the blood means that the liver, fat cells and muscles absorb and store it. The liver, because it receives most of the blood draining from the gut, plays a major role in regulating the storage and release of glucose. Some glucose is used immediately by the body but some is stored in the liver for subsequent slow release.

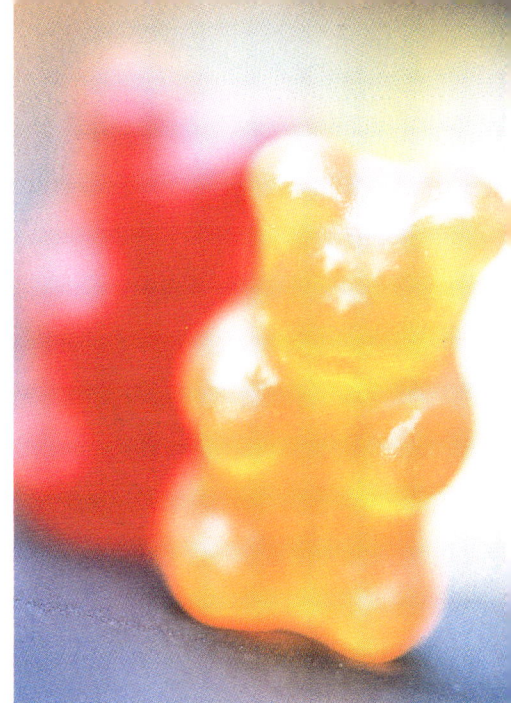

## A spoonful of uncooked vegetable oil

Ideally, simply cut out these products altogether. Give up sugar, sweetened foods and all animal fats. To flavour your meals, use just one spoonful of uncooked vegetable oil per meal. When you return to normal eating, be on the lookout for hidden sugar and fat. Cooked meats, for instance, contain large amounts of lipids. Ready meals also contain some, as well as more sugar and salt than you might expect. Read the labels carefully to avoid being caught out.

### KEY FACTS

* Before starting the detox itself, give your body some respite by avoiding all foods that foul it up and that it can well do without.

* First, cut out animal fats and refined sugars.

* Keep up this good habit after you've finished your detox programme.

## 04 make good use of aromatic herbs

Nature is a marvellous provider. It gives us aromatic herbs to flavour our food and delight our taste buds, and, what is more, it has ensured they have therapeutic, cleansing properties, too. So don't hesitate; use as many different kinds of fresh herbs as you like!

### A good habit to adopt… and maintain!

As every good chef knows, seasoning is essential when you're cooking. During your detox programme, learn how to use plenty of herbs, and continue to do so later. Aromatic herbs enable you to eat delicious – and healthy – dishes without using fatty, over-rich or sweetened ingredients. What's more, if you choose them correctly, they will help with the removal of toxins from your body.

### ●●● DID YOU KNOW?

> You can cook some aromatic herbs, such as thyme and rosemary, without diminishing their beneficial properties. Because of their thick, woody fibres, they release their active components slowly during cooking, so use them when steaming or marinating food, or when making soups.

> More delicate, leafy herbs, such as chives, parsley and basil, should be added after cooking. By doing this their aroma and beneficial qualities are not lost.

You can mix several herbs or use just one. If you choose the first approach, make sure you combine flavours that complement each other, and use herbs with similar medicinal properties to benefit one particular organ. At your next meal, you can use herbs that will help a different organ to function more efficiently.

## Some examples

**Basil** is very good for the digestion. In particular, it helps the stomach to break down food, enabling the body to absorb nutrients more efficiently, without allowing waste matter to accumulate.

**Chives** also help digestion, this time by calming upset stomachs and encouraging a healthy expulsion of wind.

**Parsley** is very rich in vitamin C, which is essential for general health and fitness, but also stimulates the kidneys and increases urine flow.

**Rosemary** is a must! It stimulates the whole body, improves digestion and helps to eliminate waste matter that has accumulated in the lungs.

**Thyme** cleans the respiratory tract and improves digestion.

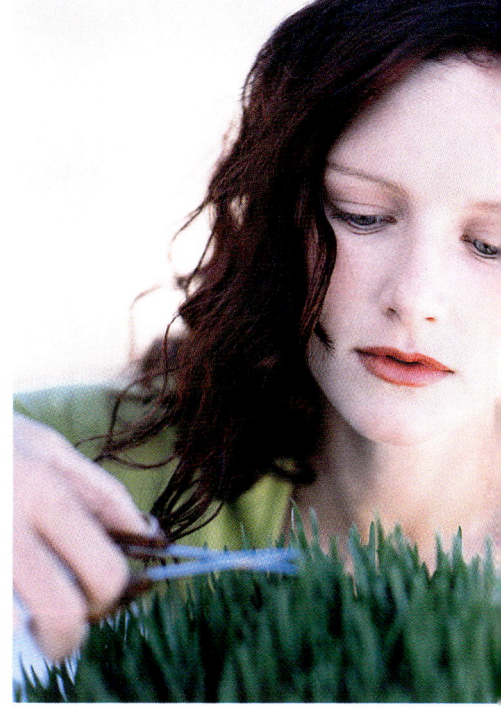

KEY FACTS

* Aromatic herbs help improve the flavour of food and aid digestion.

* Some herbs also help the excretory system to dispose of toxins.

* Thyme, rosemary, basil, parsley and chives all contribute to good health.

There's no point cleansing your body if you're going to continue to harm it in other ways. Your detox programme won't be effective unless you give up some bad habits… and the worst of all habits is smoking. Unfortunately, as any smoker will tell you, giving up is not the easiest thing to do.

## 05 you must give up smoking!

### Extremely harmful

As everyone knows, smoking damages your health in myriad ways. Cigarettes, cigars and pipe tobacco are all dangerous, although in varying degrees, and cause damage that is sometimes irreversible. A lungful of cigarette smoke contains poisonous nicotine and carbon monoxide, as well as tar, which is almost impossible for the body to excrete. Each of these three components of tobacco smoke harms the body and reduces its

● ● ● DID YOU KNOW?

> Many people trying to give up smoking worry about gaining weight, and it's true that tobacco affects the metabolism and reduces appetite.

> When we give up smoking, we use up energy more slowly and feel hunger more keenly. Also, of course, we like to snack simply because we miss having something – formerly a cigarette – in our mouth.

efficiency. Tar damages the delicate lining of the airways in the lung, making the smoker susceptible to chest infections and lung cancer in the long term, as well as to other cancers, such as of the larynx. Carbon monoxide binds to red blood cells and reduces their efficiency in carrying oxygen, while nicotine accelerates the heart rate and increases blood pressure.

The lungs, polluted by these poisons, struggle to perform their excretory functions. Consequently, other toxins, unconnected with cigarettes, are not removed effectively. A vicious circle!

## Help is at hand – with will-power!

Smoking is particularly dangerous if you've been smoking for a long time and started when young. Yet, however deeply ingrained, you must stop the habit if your body is to be detoxed. Numerous methods to help you give up are available, but nothing will work unless you are determined to do it. If you are in the right frame of mind, you may find one or a combination of the following useful: sophrology will help break the psychological addiction; acupuncture and auriculotherapy will act on the energy flow to help the body get rid of poisons; plants will help strengthen the body; homeopathy will help it regain its harmony. If all else fails, nicotine-replacement gum, patches and inhalers can be bought over the counter or prescribed by your doctor.

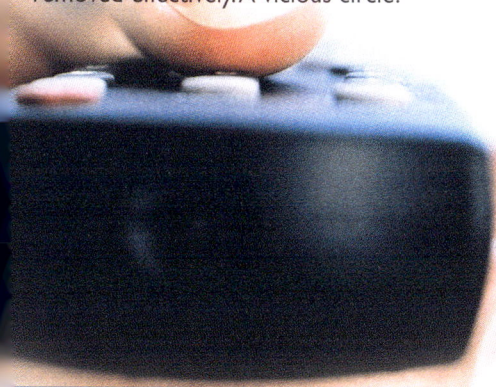

> To avoid piling on the pounds, don't snack on sweet foods during the first few weeks. Instead, choose raw vegetables, lean ham or small cubes of chicken. When you've made it through the first three or four weeks, you'll be in a better position to start dieting to get back to your old weight.

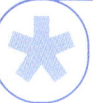

### KEY FACTS

* Tobacco damages your health in a great many ways.

* In each mouthful of cigarette smoke you inhale nicotine, carbon monoxide and tar.

* Numerous methods to help you give up smoking exist.

## 06
## cut down on coffee and alcohol

When you're tired, coffee and alcohol can give you a little energy boost. The drawback of using these stimulants, though, is that the boost is short-lived, and then you're back to square one. In fact, you're worse off, because your body has just absorbed another load of useless waste.

### Stealthy enemies

When drunk in excess, alcohol and coffee are harmful to your health and are, in effect, poisoning your body with toxins. Of course, a cup of coffee after lunch or a few glasses of good red wine with dinner won't do much harm. However, before we realize it, we're drinking too much of them every day out of habit. Coffee increases the heart rate and blood pressure, forcing the body to go

### ●●● DID YOU KNOW?

> Wine is the best form of alcohol to drink as it has several beneficial properties. Good-quality red wine contains tannins, vitamins and, most importantly, antioxidants such as polyphenols. These reduce the degenerative effects of free radicals, unstable atoms naturally produced by cell metabolism. An excess of them accelerates the ageing process.

> It is well known that excess alcohol consumption contributes to heart disease, but when drunk in small

into overdrive. It also contains several toxins that are difficult to eliminate. Alcohol affects digestion and makes immediate demands on the liver.

## Arabica and red wine

Avoid coffee and alcohol completely during your detox programme itself. Afterwards, you can drink them again, because it's counter-productive to deny yourself every pleasure, but keep within reasonable limits.

Choose arabica coffee, as it contains less caffeine than robusta, and drink no more than one or two small cups a day.

As far as alcohol is concerned, avoid spirits, aperitifs, sweet liqueurs and beer. Instead, drink wine, preferably red. The generally accepted safe limits are two glasses of wine per day for women and three glasses for men, but remember to have one or two drink-free days each week.

quantiies red wine may actually offer some protection against this condition. All of the benefits seem to be gained from just the first glass or two of the day, though; thereafter, the detrimental effects far outweigh the positive ones.

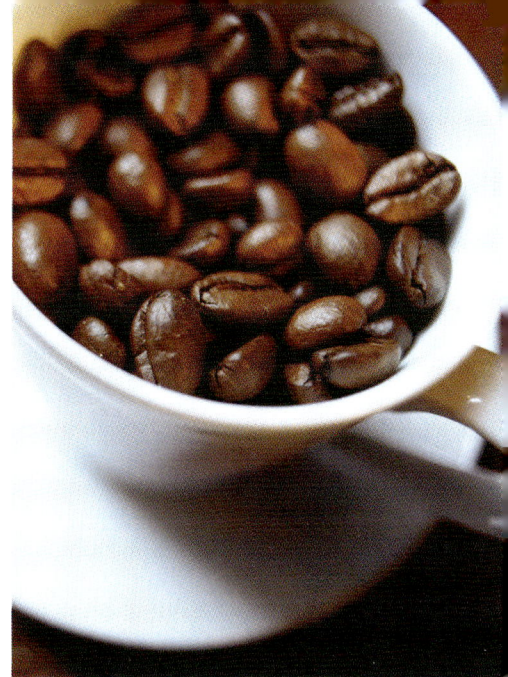

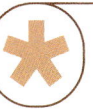

KEY FACTS

* Alcohol and coffee are stimulants and it's easy to get into the habit of drinking them every day.

* During your detox programme, give them up completely.

* Afterwards, choose arabica coffee and red wine but always in moderation.

# 07 give up animal products

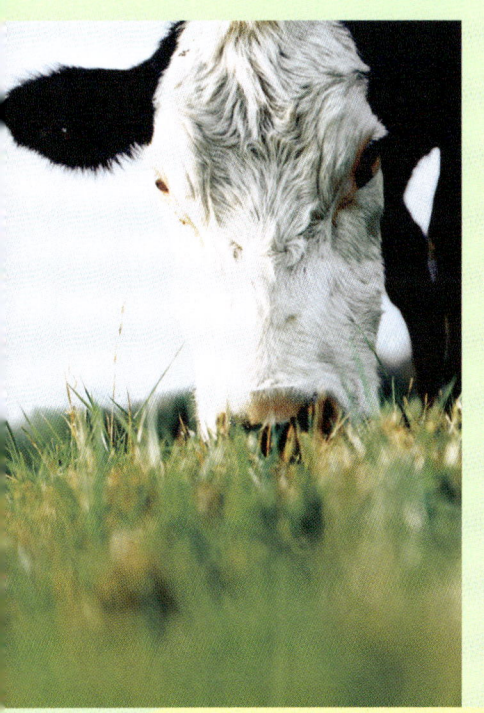

Even if you have no intention of becoming a vegetarian, you must learn to do without meat and fish completely for several days in order to give your body a rest.

### DID YOU KNOW?

> Your body won't come to any harm if it goes without animal proteins for a week or two, especially as cereals also contain proteins. However, to be effective, a cereal product must be combined with a legume vegetable at the same meal.
> Beans and wheat, lentils and rice, couscous and chickpeas: these are common combinations in poor countries, where animal proteins are in short supply and are very expensive.

## More and more toxins

Proteins are vital. Without them, the body's tissues could not grow or be repaired. Mostly found in animal products, which are the most nutritionally complete, they are broken down in the gut to form amino acids, which are then absorbed so the body can create new proteins to maintain bodily growth and repair.

However, eating too much protein leads to the creation of various forms of waste material that need to be excreted. Adults require about 65gm (2¼oz) of protein per day, and there's no evidence to suggest that consuming any more is beneficial. Although surplus amino acids may be used as a source of energy, the nitrogen molecules they contain have to be excreted as urea by the kidneys. So the more protein you consume, the harder your kidneys have to work. Foods rich in nucleic acid, such as cod roe or sweetbreads, cause overproduction of uric acid, which may lead to gout. Diets high in animal protein tend to be low in fibre but high in fat. Lack of fibre predisposes the body to constipation while too much fat leads to dyspepsia (indigestion).

## Phase them out

First, you need to give up meat. Over the course of a week, eat it twice at most. You can substitute fish, but don't eat more than one meal a day containing protein. After the first week, stop eating meat altogether and have fish only every other day. Then start to cut out all animal products. By the end of the next week completely eliminate them from your diet. A week without animal products is enough to give your excretory organs a good rest. Replace them with fruit and vegetables that cleanse the system (see Tips 14 and 15). After a week, gradually reintroduce animal products into your diet but limit them to one meal a day.

> Remember, though, that animal products (eggs and dairy, as well as fish and meat) provide nutrients that a vegan diet does not, including iron, vitamin B12, vitamin D and vitamin A, and if you go on this diet long term you will need food supplements.

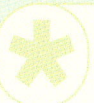

KEY FACTS

∗ Eating too much meat produces many toxins.

∗ To give your system a rest, train yourself to eat smaller and smaller amounts of meat and fish until you can go without them completely for a week, or even two.

## 08 eat more raw food

We should eat at least two portions of raw food per meal. Cooking changes the chemical structure of food and can leach out nutrients and sometimes create new toxins. Try to eat plenty of raw food.

### Heat is damaging

Raw, natural, preferably organic foodstuffs have specific chemical compositions and structures. As soon as you heat them, their composition is changed, sometimes for the worse. Fierce cooking methods, such as frying and grilling,

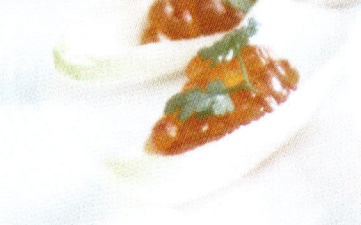

●●● DID YOU KNOW?

> You'll gradually notice that raw food has richer and more subtle tastes and flavours than cooked food.
> This is because raw food retains all its natural chemical components, many of which can be lost when food is cooked.

> Raw fruit and vegetables improve bowel movements, making it easier to eliminate toxins. This is due to the large amount of fibre in raw food. Fibre is less effective when it has been cooked (see Tip 18).

also create new substances that don't exist when the food is in its raw state. The well-grilled outer part of a lamb chop cooked over a wood fire, for instance, contains potentially carcinogenic substances.

Furthermore, while potentially dangerous substances are created, cooking foodstuffs at over 70°C means that some beneficial vitamins and minerals are lost. Boiling vegetables and throwing away the cooking water is a first-class way of reducing their vitamin C content. In addition to being packed with vitamins, raw foodstuffs provide plenty of roughage. This helps to keep the digestive system healthy and counteracts constipation. Cooking greatly reduces or almosy wholly eliminates the roughage found in most raw food. However, you should be prepared for the effects of increasing your intake of raw food. If you are used to a low-fibre diet, you will suffer less wind and bloating by increasing the fibre in your diet gradually.

## Raw food at every meal

The most suitable raw foods to eat are fruit and vegetables. To help your body cleanse itself, give it more of them.

Eat at least two portions of raw food at every meal (two portions of vegetables or one of vegetable and one of fruit). Twice a week, have a meal consisting of nothing but raw food. Food that cannot be eaten raw should be steamed or cooked over a low heat.

> Do note that this high roughage diet is not suitable for young children, who require a diet high in calories, iron and vitamins.

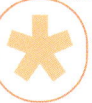 KEY FACTS

* Eat two pieces of raw food per meal, and twice a week eat an entirely raw meal.

* Fruit and vegetables contain fibre, minerals and vitamins, but some of these are destroyed by cooking. When you have to cook food, do so gently.

## 09
## in springtime try a strawberry diet

It's now time to go a step further. One good option is a fruit monodiet. Natural medicine practitioners often consider this the best way to detox. The principle is simple: you eat just one type of fruit and nothing else for three days. It's guaranteed to work.

### Just one type of fruit

If detox has a season, it's got to be the spring. At this time of year the body naturally goes into a cleansing phase to rid itself of the toxins accumulated during the winter, when we generally take less exercise (it's too wet and windy to go for a jog) and eat more (just think of Christmas time).

To help your body to cleanse itself, try a monodiet of strawberries. If you're

● ● ● DID YOU KNOW?

> Don't dive straight into a monodiet. First reduce the amount of 'heavy' foods you eat by gradually cutting out sugars, fats, dairy products, animal proteins and cereals.
> When your diet comprises only fruit and vegetables, choose the one that best suits your taste, digestion and lifestyle, then eat nothing but that for one day.
> The first time you attempt a monodiet, it's best to restrict yourself to that single day, but the next time you try it you can go for two days,

allergic to them, try another fruit with the same purifying qualities (peach, kiwi fruit, etc.) or a vegetable (such as celery or asparagus).

## Your liver loves strawberries!

A monodiet allows your system almost complete rest. The digestion and absorption of food is reduced to the barest minimum, which enables the excretory organs to embark upon a big clear-out. If, in addition, you choose to eat a plant with cleansing, purifying properties, that's even better. Strawberries are very rich in vitamin C and mineral salts, and they are a delicious way to enjoy these nutrients. Also, they assist in the flushing out of toxins, particularly uric acid, which helps to combat illnesses associated with 'overwork', such as high blood pressure, and certain forms of rheumatism caused by an accumulation of toxins in the joints.

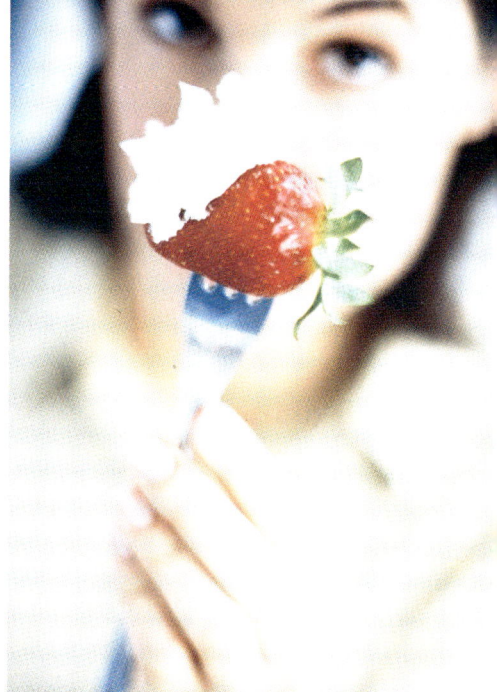

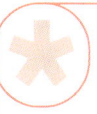 KEY FACTS

* Nothing rests the body and helps it to cleanse itself as well as a monodiet.

* Try a strawberry monodiet in the spring: it's the ideal way to stimulate the liver.

* You need to phase in the week before a monodiet, and phase out the week after.

# 10 in summer try a cherry diet

For your summer monodiet, you may want to substitute cherries for strawberries. This delicious fruit has exceptional cleansing qualities. It also contains minerals and is a good source of energy.

**Diuretic and laxative qualities** Cherries are sweeter than strawberries, so, unsurprisingly, they contain more calories. They also contain large amounts of potassium, magnesium and calcium, and some vitamin C. As their flesh is 80 per cent water, they cleanse the kidneys. Since they possess both diuretic and slightly laxative qualities, but also the vital minerals listed above, they are an excellent choice for a monodiet. There are plenty of different varieties, so you can try different flavours and textures to make your diet more interesting and enjoyable: all the varieties have virtually the same qualities.

**Not a fan of cherries?** Try a monodiet of melons or raspberries instead. Melon has similar diuretic and laxative properties to those of cherries, while raspberries are effective diuretics. They are also thought to stimulate blood circulation.

● ● ● DID YOU KNOW?

> When on a monodiet, you must eat your chosen fruit or vegetable without any sweetener or flavouring – so no sugar on your cherries or cream on your strawberries, and no port with your melon. Most people find that this is easier to do with fruit than with vegetables.

KEY FACTS

∗ Cherries have diuretic and laxative properties.

∗ Eat them without any sweetener or flavouring.

∗ You could also use melons and raspberries for your monodiet.

# 11 in autumn try a grape diet

In autumn, grapes become the stars of the monodiet. Whether red or white, they're great for cleansing the kidneys and intestines.

**Carbohydrates and mineral salts** Grapes are a good source of energy as they contain many different carbohydrates in high concentration. They are also rich in minerals, particularly potassium, magnesium and phosphorus. They don't contain much vitamin C, but the little they have is combined with other substances in such a way that it is easily absorbed. They're also a good source of vitamin B. All this means that at the end of your diet, you'll not only be cleansed but full of energy!

**Helping digestion and stimulating the kidneys** Grapes help at all stages of the digestive process: they stimulate the muscles of the stomach walls, promote bowel movements and accelerate the expulsion of intestinal toxins. They also help the kidneys: being rich in potassium with a small amount of sodium, they have powerful diuretic qualities. Finally, they may help to reduce acidity in the urine and the level of uric acid in the blood.

### DID YOU KNOW?

> Choose organic grapes whenever possible.
> Rinse them quickly but thoroughly, and don't leave them to soak in water or they will lose some of their nutrients.
> Don't keep them for too long before eating them.

### KEY FACTS

* Grapes have purifying, laxative, diuretic and energy-giving qualities.

* After your grape diet, you'll be cleansed and will have enough energy to face the winter.

* Choose organic grapes, don't rinse them too much and eat them when they are fresh.

# 12 fasting? – take great care

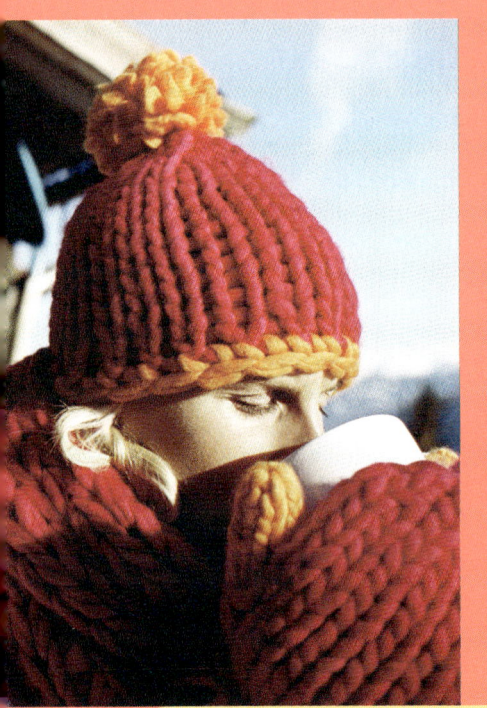

To rest your system, you can deprive your body of all food. This is effective, but it must be done with great care because it's a risky strategy. You need to reduce your food intake gradually and fast for only a very limited period.

### DID YOU KNOW?

> When fasting, you lose the sensation of hunger after one day. That's why experienced fasters can carry on for more than three days. However, don't try this the first time you fast.

> Rest as much as you can. Don't plan anything requiring intense effort and try to avoid losing your temper. If you've never practised relaxation or meditation before, this is a good time to start: you can rest your mind and emotions as well as your body.

## To be done in moderation

The principle of fasting couldn't be easier: you simply stop eating. It's the most extreme method of giving the digestive system a break and allowing the body to cleanse itself. During a fast, the body burns up its reserves of energy, mostly in the form of fat. After all, that's what it's there for: it's the human body's evolutionary safeguard against starvation. Many toxins are stored in fatty tissues, so when the fat is broken down these are released and can be expelled.

However, fasting can be dangerous if not carried out carefully. While the breaking down of fat is a good aspect of autolysis – the term for when the body draws on its reserves of energy during fasting – there is a downside. The body gets energy wherever it can, so muscle tissue is broken down alongside fat; and stocks of vitamins and minerals are depleted, too. This is why a fast should be preceded by careful preparation and must not last too long. Use it sparingly.

## A well-organized fasting programme

- The first three days: gradually cut out proteins (meat, fish, dairy products), followed by fats (butter, oil).
- The next three days: eat only fruit and vegetables.
- Now you're ready to fast: for the next three days, consume nothing but water, vegetable stock (without the vegetables) and calming or cleansing herbal teas (lime tree, vervain, lemon balm, fennel, artichoke, mallow, marsh mallow). You might not last for three days, but try to go for at least twenty-four hours without food.
- Gradually start eating again, starting with cooked fruit and vegetables, then uncooked ones, cereals, uncooked oils and finally proteins and cooked fatty foods.

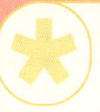

### KEY FACTS

* Fasting is an effective technique but carries risks.

* Follow a fasting programme spread over about two weeks, and rest physically and mentally while fasting.

* Before embarking on a fast consult your doctor if you have any health concerns.

> If you are on medication or have any health concerns, take advice from your doctor before embarking on a fast.

# 13 fruit and veg are good for the liver

Nature has provided us with plants that cleanse the liver and help remove toxins that accumulate there. If you feel a little sluggish, make sure that you eat artichokes, black radishes, dandelion and pineapples regularly.

## Artichokes are a must

The artichoke is rich in vitamin A and potassium. It is a flower bud belonging to the thistle family and has been used for centuries in French traditional folk medicine to improve the functioning of the liver and protect it from infection. It contains plenty of potassium and a good quantity of fibre, but not many calories. It can be eaten raw or cooked (boiled or

### ●●● DID YOU KNOW?

> Why not eat more exotic fruit?
> The pineapple contains enzymes that help digestion, particularly the digestion of proteins. One of them, bromelain, is especially effective in breaking down proteins.

> Papain, in the papaya fruit, has similar properties.
> Mangoes help to digest fatty foods, particularly the combinations of proteins and lipids found in marbled red meat.

steamed), with a dressing of olive oil and cider vinegar or lemon juice.

Artichoke leaves are also beneficial. If you buy small artichokes that have a piece of stalk and some leaves attached, cook everything and keep the broth so that you can drink a glass at the beginning of the meal. It doesn't taste great, but it certainly does you good!

## Root crops with medicinal properties

Black radishes come a close second to artichokes as liver purifiers. They promote both the secretion and the expulsion of bile, as well as the regeneration of liver cells. They may be eaten on their own or as part of a salad, and can be diced or grated. They have a strong flavour, which can be quite pleasant once you have acquired it. However, if you don't like the taste, black radish juice is available in phials. Pink radishes are less effective but do still stimulate the liver.

Carrots help the bile to carry waste products away from the liver by making it more fluid.

Finally, try some dandelions when they are in season, because they are excellent for cleansing the liver and the biliary system. Their bitter, rather strange taste can be made more palatable by eating them with slices of apple and a sauce of walnut oil or fruit vinegar (raspberry, fig, pear).

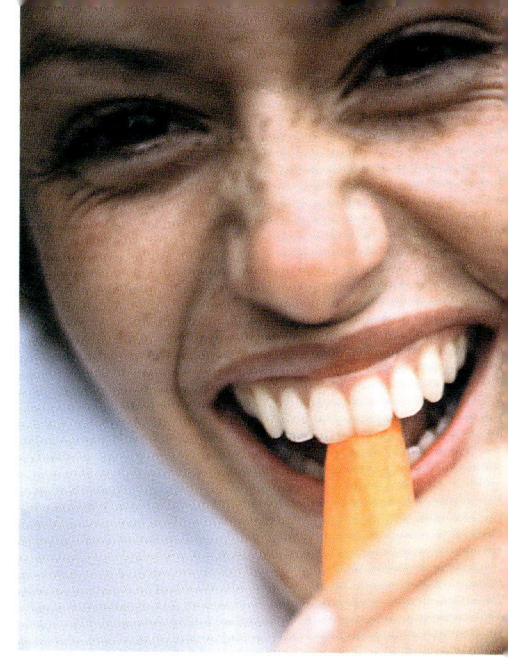

### KEY FACTS

* The artichoke is rich in vitamin A and potassium.

* Black radishes and, to a lesser extent, pink radishes have a cleansing effect on both the gall-bladder and the liver.

* Some exotic fruits can help improve digestion.

# 14 fruit and veg are good for the kidneys

**Some plants – for instance, asparagus, beetroot, celery and cucumber – have powerful diuretic qualities. They can help the kidneys to eliminate waste from the body and also help them to purify themselves.**

## A vegetable with two vital functions

The diuretic properties of asparagus have been well known for many hundreds of years. Many of its constituents, such as asparagin, stimulate the production of urine. As a result, asparagus was prescribed in traditional folk medicine as a treatment for fluid retention and high blood pressure. Asparagin has another beneficial quality, too: it accelerates the production of new cells. Asparagus,

### ●●● DID YOU KNOW?

> Eating plenty of citrus fruit provides numerous health benefits.
> Grapefruit contains a lot of potassium and, therefore, accelerates urine production.
> Lemons purify the blood and speed up its circulation, which helps to stimulate the removal of waste by the kidneys.

> The same is true of kumquats, which contain large amounts of vitamins and minerals in the flesh, and in the skin, which should be eaten, too.

therefore, performs two vital detoxification functions: it helps excrete waste and promotes the renewal of bodily organs. Asparagus, whether green or white, may be steamed or boiled and flavoured with vegetable oil and a little lemon juice. The flavour can be enhanced by varying the quantity of oil used.

## A salad of cucumber, celery or beetroot

Although not as potent as asparagus, cucumber also has diuretic, cleansing qualities, because of its very high water content. Don't dry it, as you'll lose the benefit of the numerous substances contained in its fluid if you do.

You can also help your kidney function, and that other excretory organs, by regularly eating beetroot, a vegetable that is low in calories, despite its high sugar content. Another of its virtues, and a considerable one, is that it lowers the level of bad cholesterol in the blood. Don't be alarmed by one of its completely harmless side-effects: if you eat a lot of beetroot, your urine might well be stained pink.

Finally, don't forget celery. It cleans waste matter from the blood and also helps the kidneys to eliminate it. You can eat as much of it as you like, either raw or cooked.

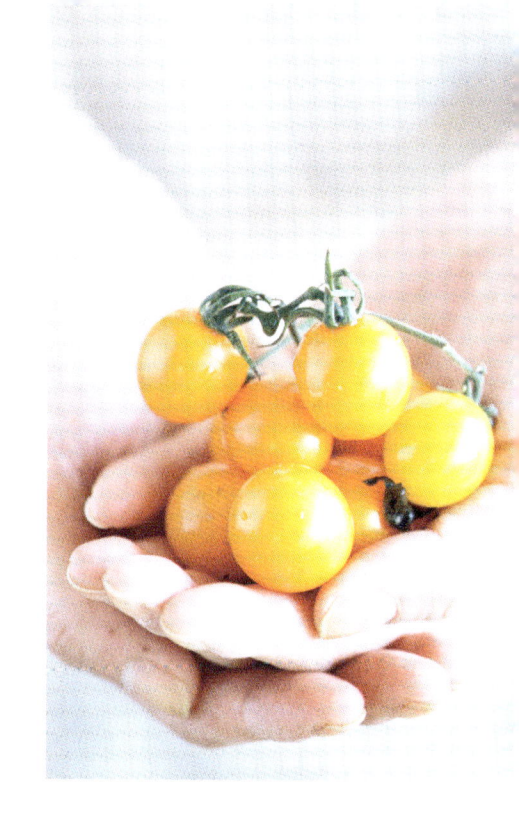

### KEY FACTS

* Asparagus is the diuretic vegetable *par excellence*.

* Cucumber, beetroot and celery are also excellent in helping the body to eliminate waste.

* Citrus fruits are very useful in this respect, too.

# 15 fruit and veg for healthy bowels

**No detox programme will succeed if you suffer from constipation. Sluggish intestines lead to a build up of toxins that infiltrate the rest of the body. To avoid this stealthy form of poisoning, eat figs, leeks and prunes.**

### Eat prunes and drink prune juice

Many people remember being given prunes as a natural alternative to laxatives when they were children. But, of course, adults can benefit from them too. They are packed with dietary fibre, which increases stool bulk, and complex sugars, which are better for the digestive system. As a result, food is processed more quickly from the small to the large intestine, where digestive bacteria are

### ●●● DID YOU KNOW?

> Figs also have an excellent cleansing effect on the intestines, thanks to a substance called mucin.

> Just like prunes, figs increase the volume of stools and accelerate their removal.

> They may be eaten fresh or dried, cooked or raw, and even drunk as a syrup.

more numerous and more active, and, therefore, work more effectively. Also, muscular contractions are stronger and more frequent, so that stools are expelled more easily and more rapidly from the large intestine. Finally, prunes contain a large amount of the laxative sugar sorbitol. As they boast all of these properties, use prunes with discretion: eating too many can give you diarrhoea and/or colic.

You can eat prunes raw or stew them. Prune juice is also very effective, particularly if it is taken on an empty stomach and at body temperature.

## Just like a cleaning brush

The leek is a fantastic vegetable for encouraging bowel movements. It contains long fibres, mucilage and cellulose, and acts on the intestines like a brush. Impurities are picked up as the fibres pass through and are later expelled with the fibres themselves.

Leeks are usually boiled or steamed, and seasoned with olive oil and lemon. They may also be made into a soup. When cooked in this way, they will help to cleanse both your kidneys and your liver.

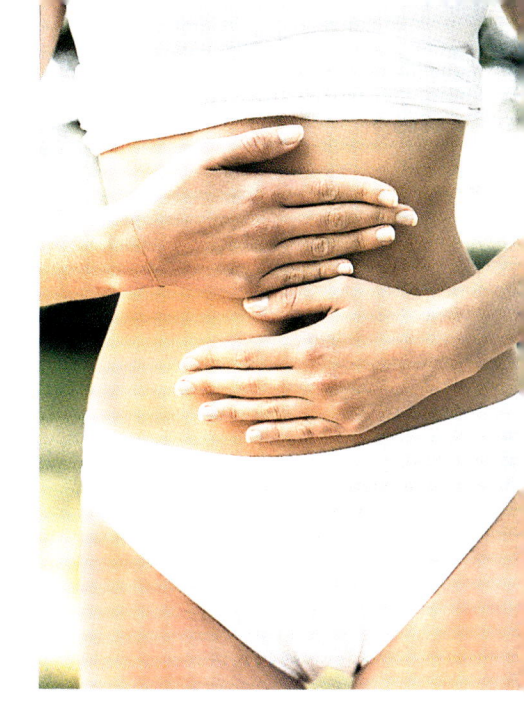

### KEY FACTS

* Prunes have been a well-known cure for constipation for centuries.

* Figs have a similar effect.

* Because of their long fibres, leeks act like a gentle brush, collecting impurities and pulling them along to be expelled from the body.

# 16 try a course of lemon juice

**The lemon has amazing powers. High in potassium, calcium and, of course, vitamin C, it increases blood flow and cleanses the lymphatic system.**

**Acids to combat acids** Contrary to a misconception held by many people, eating a lemon causes little or no stomach acidity. Its acids, particularly citric acid, are broken down during various stages of digestion and then form alkaline substances. So, instead of increasing the level of uric acid, the lemon helps to reduce it. It's therefore perfectly safe to eat or drink, unless you have an ulcer or have been diagnosed as suffering from hyperacidity.

**A wonderful tonic** Lemons are highly recommended in a detoxing programme. They stimulate the kidneys and, what's more, being rich in chlorine and potassium, they increase the volume of urine produced. They are also carminative (help to relieve colic), stimulate the bronchial tubes and are tonics for the stomach, the liver and the veins. Finally, they are rich in revitalizing vitamin C and mineral salts.

### ●●● DID YOU KNOW?

> Every morning, drink some lemon juice mixed with some low-mineral water. Begin by using just half a lemon, then one, two and so on until you are drinking the juice of six lemons. Then reverse the process until you are back to half a lemon a day.

### KEY FACTS

* Lemons stimulate the kidneys, the liver and the lungs, and are revitalizing.

* A course of lemon juice treatment lasts for two weeks.

# 17 drink clay

**A short course of clay-water milk at the beginning of each of the four seasons will cleanse you from top to toe. Clay compresses and poultices are also useful.**

## From ancient Egypt to the present day

Clay has been used therapeutically since the days of ancient Egypt and all over the world. Thick and sticky when wet, powdery when dry, it is formed from the slow decomposition of certain crystalline rocks, such as granite. One of its chief characteristics is extraordinary absorbency: if it comes into contact with toxins, they will be bed by the clay and may then be expelled.

## A daily regime

Every evening, pour a teaspoonful of powdered clay into a glass of mineral water, stir and leave to settle overnight. The next morning, before you've eaten anything, stir the mixture again and drink it. If you can't bear the taste of the clay, drink the water without stirring it in the morning. Once inside the digestive tract, the clay will absorb all the waste matter and ensure that it's expelled.

### ● ● ● DID YOU KNOW?

> If you can't bear to drink clay-water milk, roll some clay into little balls, half a centimetre in diameter. Mix them with water to make quite a thick paste and let them dry. Every morning, before you have eaten anything, swallow three of the little balls with a large glass of water.

### KEY FACTS

* Clay possesses very strong powers of absorption, which enables it to collect waste matter and expel it.

* Regularly take a course of clay-water milk.

* Alternatively, prepare some small balls of clay to swallow like tablets.

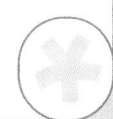

# 18 eat plenty of fibre

Fibre is a component of food and yet we are unable to digest almost all of it. But it is still absolutely vital to our well-being. Dietary fibre is crucial to the smooth working of our digestive system. Without it, we would suffer pain, constipation and often piles.

## Soluble and insoluble fibre

There are two kinds of dietary fibre: indigestible and digestible. The first, known as 'insoluble', are indispensable to the smooth functioning of the intestines. Firstly, they slow down the movement of the mass of semi-digested food from the stomach into the small intestine, giving the various gastric juices time to do their jobs properly. Once they've helped in this way, they then facilitate the rapid

### ●●● DID YOU KNOW?

> Fruit and vegetables are good sources of fibre, although they are less effective than those found in cereals and pulses. Eat at least three foods from these four categories at every meal.

> In addition to all its other advantages, fibre fills you up rapidly, so you will be able to reduce your food intake without feeling hungry.

movement of the mass towards the large intestine. This reduces the risk of fermentation and poisoning.

'Soluble' fibres are partially digested. They help to slow the absorption of sugars and fats into the bloodstream and thus reduce peak levels of glucose in the blood and insulin release from the pancreas. This helps to minimize variations of glucose level in the bloodstream and so addresses associated symptoms such as headaches, dizziness and sugar cravings. Also, soluble fibres bind on to blood cholesterol, allowing some of it to be expelled in the stool.

## A gift from the plant world to keep us healthy

These vital fibres are found only in the plant world, in fruit, vegetables, cereals and pulses. The fibre from wholemeal cereals (wheat, rice, quinoa, etc.) and pulses (lentils, beans, chickpeas, etc.) are the most effective. The fibres are usually to be found in the outer membrane of plants. Unfortunately, this is precisely where chemicals used in intensive farming, such as pesticides and fertilizers, are most concentrated. If you want to benefit from dietary fibre without consuming the chemicals too, it's best to eat organically grown cereals and pulses.

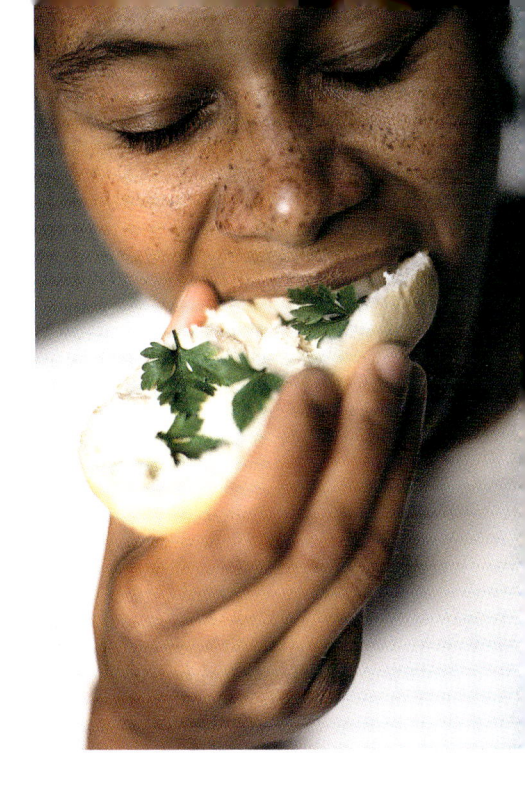

### KEY FACTS

* Dietary fibre is vital to the smooth functioning of the intestines.

* It improves digestion and removes certain harmful substances such as cholesterol.

* It is found only in plants: fruit, vegetables, cereals and pulses.

# 19 drink tea, then more tea

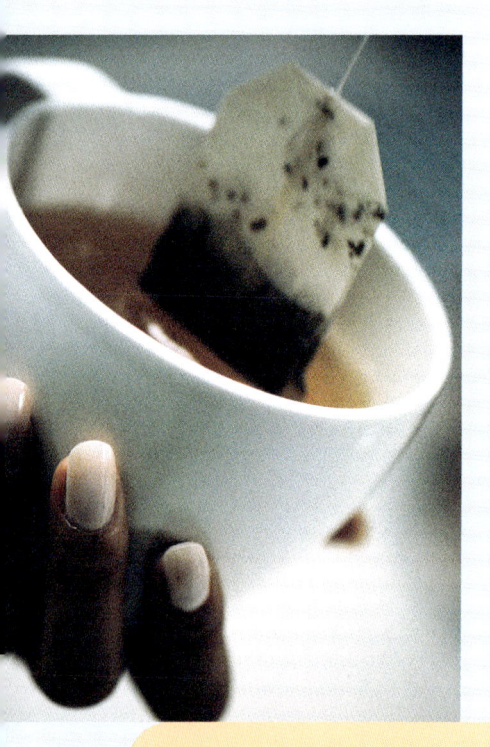

As almost everyone knows, tea is diuretic. However, this drink, popular all over the world, has other virtues, too. In particular, it combats the damaging effects of free radicals.

### DID YOU KNOW?
> The medicinal properties of tea differ according to colour.

> Green tea is dried after it has been picked and possesses more tannin. Consequently, it works more effectively against free radicals.

## Tiny time bombs

Tea is drunk almost everywhere at breakfast time. An average English adult drinks two thousand cups of it each year! And that's fine, because tea is genuinely medicinal and possesses many beneficial qualities. First, it provides exceptional protection against free radicals, which accelerate the ageing of our cells and therefore our organs. Strictly speaking, free radicals are neither waste matter nor toxins, but a detox programme should nevertheless aim to do something about them. These products of cell metabolism are unstable atoms or molecules that exist for only a fraction of a second but still have the time to cause irreversible damage. They attack cell walls and prevent them from being properly supplied with food; they also damage the cell core and can even distort DNA. We each produce several billion free radicals every second and they cause our bodies to deteriorate slowly but surely.

## A friend to the kidneys

Tea contains large quantities of flavonoids and tannins. Like the polyphenols in grapes, these chemicals protect us from free radicals. In addition, tea is very diuretic: it stimulates the filtering activity of the kidneys and increases urine volume. It also helps the process of digestion.

Tea is very rich in theine (a substance very similar to caffeine), theobromine and theophylline, all of which stimulate the central nervous system. This is why some people suffer from insomnia if they drink too much tea. If you're not one of them, you may safely drink several cups a day. Otherwise, just drink a cup at breakfast time and another during your mid-morning break.

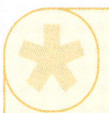

> Black tea is fermented in humid conditions and has a higher flavonoid content, which makes it better for protecting the cardiovascular system.
> Both kinds of tea have the same diuretic and purifying qualities.

### KEY FACTS

* Tea protects the body from the destructive effects of free radicals.

* It is a diuretic and stimulates the central nervous system.

* Green and black tea have different medicinal qualities.

# 20 don't confuse detox with slimming

During your detox programme, it's highly likely that you'll lose weight. Don't, however, think that detoxing is a slimming diet. You'll be disappointed if you do.

**Weight lost …** You'll soon see the effect of your detox programme when you step on the scales. Frequent visits to the toilet, the elimination of toxins and resting your metabolism all lead to weight loss. Depending on the individual and the rigour of the programme, you can lose anything from one to four kilos over a fortnight. But detoxing is different from slimming. When you go on a diet, you don't usually go without most foodstuffs for a short period but try, in a more sustained way, to change your eating habits.

**… and regained** Once it has been detoxed for 1–3 days, the body's functions return to normal. The muscles, which will have got smaller during the programme, return to their former size, and the body's water levels increase to normal. If you don't take the opportunity to change your eating habits, your weight will soon return to its former level too.

### ● ● ● DID YOU KNOW?

> If you want to avoid putting weight back on, you need to work out how to improve your everyday diet. A detox programme is a particularly good time to attempt this, but you should realise that it will require a long-term, ongoing effort.

### KEY FACTS

* Detoxing involves making the body undergo shortages in order to cleanse it, while a slimming diet means changing eating habits.

* Any weight lost during the detoxing programme will soon be regained unless you use this opportunity to correct your bad eating habits.

# case study

**The weight went back on but I feel so much better**

« I'd put on ten kilos, grew breathless as soon as I did anything more active than a gentle walk, I was covered in spots and always catching colds. My doctor, who's interested in complementary medicine, advised me to try a detox treatment. I didn't really understand what he meant but I took his advice: I drank clay every morning, ate plants to help the kidneys and the liver and followed a carefully programmed diet. I've no particular comments to make about the clay and the plants but the diet was hard! I had to start again from scratch several times before I managed it. I ended up going away for a fortnight to an isolated house in the country, away from temptation, worries and interruptions. I didn't think it would be, but detoxing was an amazing experience. Eating less and less, feeling the hunger pangs diminishing and then disappearing altogether, feeling my body getting lighter. At the beginning, I got some spots and my stomach felt bloated but that soon passed. I lost five kilos, which I soon put back on, but the sensation of lightness has remained! »

# 21 >>>

》 **During your detox programme,** however long it might last, your liver, kidneys, skin and lungs will have plenty of work to do. So give them some help.

》》》 To encourage your body to sweat, take hot baths and exercise. **Plants and massage** will help your liver and your kidneys. Use essential oils and take walks in the fresh air to help your lungs.

》》》》》 **And don't neglect traditional treatments.** They've proved their worth over centuries and should be just as popular today as they ever were.

# 40
## TIPS

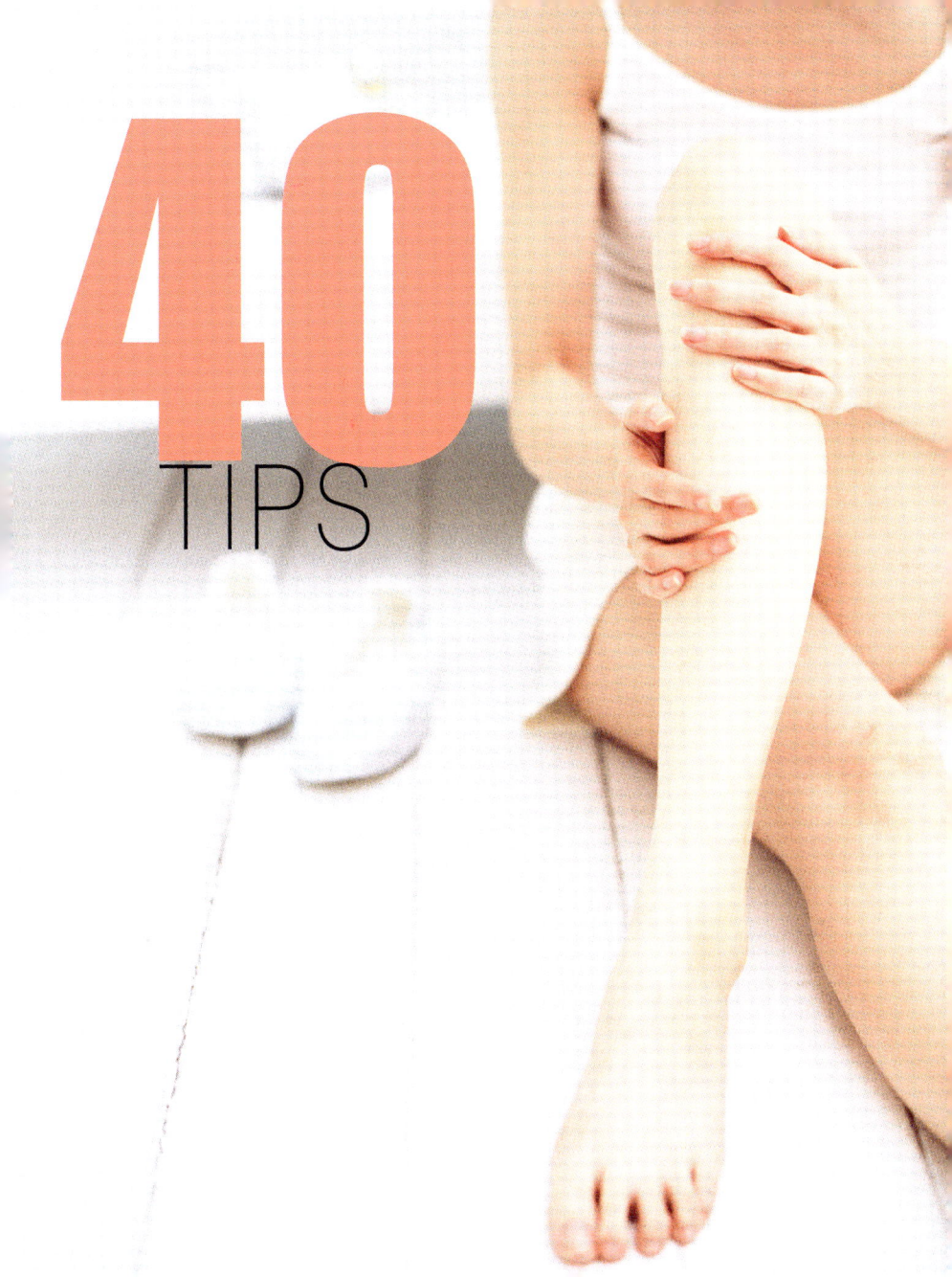

## 21 sweat it out

Sweating must never be considered as something nasty and smelly that should be avoided. It's a natural way of excreting toxins from the body. To help your skin perform this vital function, why not take a trip to the sauna or the steam room? You'll come out feeling cleansed, inside and out.

### More than just a protective wrapping

Our skin is more than just an outer membrane that protects our internal organs from the outside world. It is an organ in its own right and performs many functions, among them the secretion of hormones and breathing. Through sweating, it excretes certain forms of waste matter, including urea and uric acid, as well as salt. The sweat

### ● ● ● DID YOU KNOW?

> The steam room originated in North Africa and the Middle East. Unlike a sauna, it produces a very humid heat. Traditional steam rooms comprise several rooms, each at a different temperature, and you move from one to another as you wish. Consequently, a steam usually lasts longer than a sauna.

> Humidity and heat together soften the surface of the skin, allowing it to be thoroughly cleaned. By removing dead cells, exfoliation treatments and massage can improve skin functioning for several weeks.

glands are very similar to nephrons, the cells in the kidneys that filter out waste. Our skin is linked to thousands of kilometres of tiny blood vessels, which are often just below the surface. The blood is filtered as it makes its journey around the body and the waste is expelled through the skin's pores.

## Heat and sweat

In addition to its excretory function, sweat helps to maintain a constant body temperature. When it's hot outside, the body produces sweat to lower the internal body temperature, which is why we sweat much more in hot weather.

The sauna, which originated in the Nordic countries, is a little wooden cabin complete with a source of intense, very dry heat that stimulates perspiration and thus improves the elimination of toxins. A sauna needs to be used with care: you shouldn't stay in it for too long and you shouldn't use one at all if you suffer from high blood pressure or heart problems, however slight. Plant vapours are often diffused inside the sauna to clear the bronchial tubes.

The ideal way to use sauna is to stay in for five minutes, then take a cold shower, and afterwards rest for a quarter of an hour. Repeat the procedure two or three times.

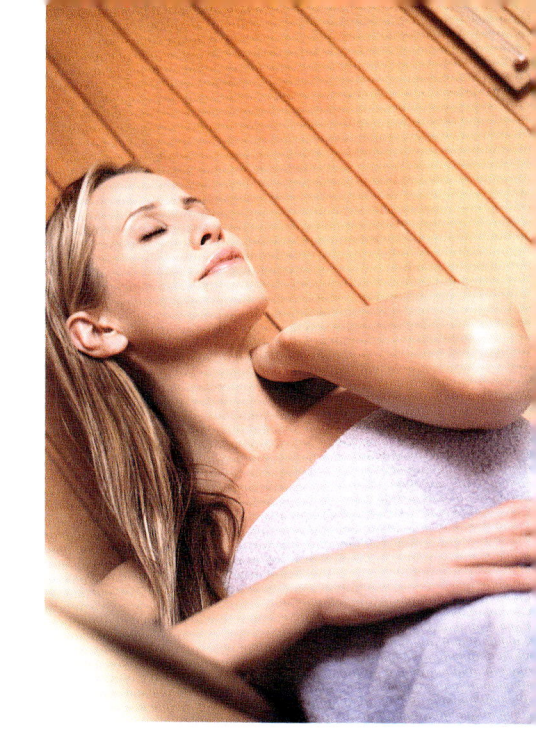

### KEY FACTS

* The skin is an organ in its own right that removes waste by means of sweat.

* Sweat helps to maintain a constant body temperature by cooling the body in hot weather.

* Saunas and steam rooms improve the elimination of toxins from the body.

## 22 get moving!

Another good way of raising a sweat is through exercise. Intense physical activity causes the body temperature to rise and accelerates the elimination of toxins. It doesn't matter which form of exercise you choose, as long as it makes you sweat.

### Rushing around makes you hot

Increased physical activity causes increased body temperature. As everyone knows, when you rush about, you get hot. There are several reasons for this. First, exercise speeds up metabolic processes throughout the body. This, in turn, causes the production of more waste matter, which is eliminated, to some extent, by respiration and, to a much larger extent, by perspiration.

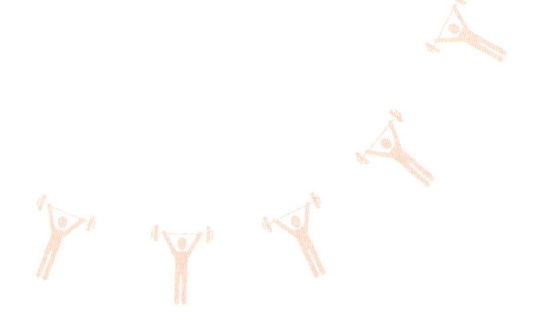

### ●●● DID YOU KNOW?

> In order to sweat more, if the weather is not too hot, wear a tracksuit, rather than stripping down to the bare essentials.

> After the session, take a shower to wash away the toxins that will have accumulated on your skin. Then treat yourself to a little rest to allow your body to recover from its exertion.

In addition, the body has to provide more energy for the muscles, particularly the cardiac muscles, to enable them to make the required effort. The use of this energy produces heat, which has to be dissipated.

## Fast and sustained effort

Sweating, therefore, performs a dual role: it regulates body temperature and eliminates the extra waste. It doesn't matter what you choose to do, as long as it requires sustained effort. Gentle activity isn't sufficient because a substantial increase in body temperature is needed. The exercise must initially be intense enough for you to break into a sweat, and you need to keep going for as long as you can (without overdoing it, of course). The aim is not to break any endurance records but just to work up a good sweat and then maintain it.

Tennis and jogging are particularly suitable, but you need to ensure you are at an adequate level of fitness before embarking upon this type of physical activity, especially if you haven't done any exercise for a long time. And be sensible in hot, humid weather as too much exercise can lead to overheating.

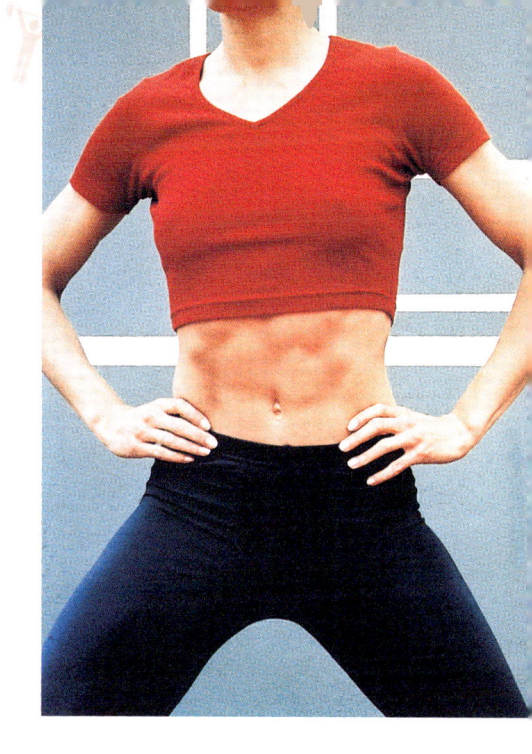

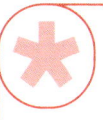

### KEY FACTS

* Intense physical activity increases body temperature and makes you sweat more.

* The effort must be sustained for long enough in order to cause a sweat.

* After the session, take a shower and allow your body to rest.

# 23 herbal teas to make you sweat

Sudorifics are plants that make you sweat more. You can use them as part of your detox programme. It's a perfectly natural method but one best reserved for a quiet day at home.

## A nice hot cup of herbal tea

Drinking a cup of hot herbal tea while lying warm in bed is another good way of getting rid of toxins. You could also place a hot-water bottle under the covers with you. Make sure, however, that you choose the right herbal tea, one infused from a sudorific medicinal herb. This means that it will naturally increase perspiration without causing any harm.

### ● ● ● DID YOU KNOW?

> Before going to bed with your herbal tea, rub your skin with a massage glove.

> The friction accelerates **blood** circulation directly under the skin and increases the amount of waste that is filtered out. After doing this, your perspiration will contain more toxins.

Elderflower is a good choice. These pretty, sweet-smelling, umbrella-shaped clusters of flowers are a traditional remedy for respiratory illnesses because they promote sweating and the elimination of toxins. But you don't need to be suffering from bronchitis to enjoy a cup of elderflower tea. Put a tablespoonful of dried flowers in a large cup of boiling water and leave to infuse for ten minutes before filtering. Drink the tea, if possible, between meals, then lie down in the warm for half an hour.

## Food for Smurfs

Many children will be familiar with the pointed, shiny sarsaparilla leaves eaten by Smurfs. However, it's not the leaves but the root of the sarsaparilla, dried and ground up, that is used in herbal medicine. Among other virtues, it's both diuretic and sudorific. Boil two tablespoonfuls of sarsaparilla root in about 500ml (1 pint) of water until roughly half of the liquid has evaporated. Filter off the remaining liquid and drink sweetened with honey (it doesn't taste too good without the honey).

You could also try lungwort. Put a tablespoonful of the plant in a large cup of boiling water and leave to infuse for ten minutes before drinking.

> The friction also removes dead cells that would otherwise impede the process of cleansing.

### KEY FACTS

* There are several different plants (elderflower, sarsaparilla and lungwort) that promote sweating.

* Rub your skin with a massage glove before drinking your herbal tea and then lie down in a warm bed for half an hour.

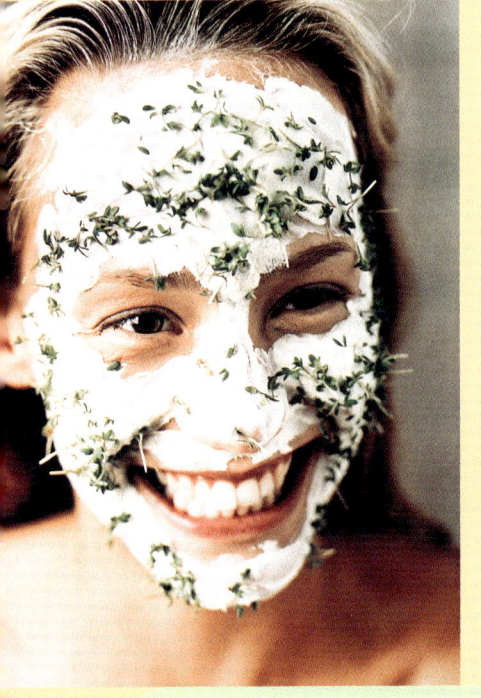

# 24 plants that are good for the skin

Your skin must be in good condition if it is to carry out its function of removing toxins from the body. A healthy skin will be more efficient than one that is greasy or dry, irritated or inflamed. Plants can be used to overcome a variety of skin complaints.

### ••• DID YOU KNOW?

> Acne is a sign that toxins are not being eliminated efficiently from the body. If it affects a large part of your body, you should consult a doctor.

> If you suffer from the odd spot from time to time, treat it with one of the following lotions:
- Infuse 50g (2oz) of saponin in 500ml (1 pint) of boiling water for around 10 minutes.

## If you have greasy skin

People with shiny, greasy skin produce an excess of sebum. This is a natural secretion that is essential to keep the skin moist. It is produced by the sebaceous glands, which are situated at the base of hair follicles. When there's too much of it, it blocks the skin's pores.

If your skin is too greasy, use a juice extractor to combine the juices of carrot, chervil, lettuce and grapefruit. This can then be used as a lotion. Apply the mixture every evening before going to bed. Once a week, using a food mixer, prepare a face mask of cucumber and fresh tomatoes; spread quite a thick layer on your skin. Let it dry, rinse off and then apply the juice lotion.

## If you have dry skin

Unsurprisingly, dry skin is the result of a shortage of sebum. Dead skin cells accumulate because sedum is not being produced in large enough quantities to remove them. The pores become blocked and the skin's cleansing ability diminishes. To treat this condition, make lily-flower oil by soaking 50g (2oz) of lily flowers in a jar of evening primrose or borage oil. Use just enough oil to cover the flowers. Put the lid on the jar and boil it in a bain-marie for two hours. Allow to cool, then filter the oil through a fine cloth and store in a cool place. Apply this oil to your face before going to bed each evening.

To make a suitable mask, choose, according to the season, either the flesh of a peach (blended in a food mixer and then spread on just as it is) or a mixture of apples and pears cooked in milk. Spread on thickly and keep it on for ten minutes before rinsing it off with cornflower or witch-hazel water.

- Boil 10g (1/3oz) of burdock, 10g of marigold and 10g of wild pansy in 500ml (1 pint) of water for around 10 minutes.

### KEY FACTS

* To eliminate waste efficiently, the skin must not be too greasy or too dry.

* If it is too dry, treat it with lily-flower oil and a peach face mask.

* Use carrot lotion and a tomato face mask if your skin is greasy.

## 25 treat yourself to lymphatic drainage

The lymphatic system is the body's main refuse collector. It picks up waste matter and transports it to the bloodstream, which then disposes of it. A specific kind of massage improves the circulation of lymph fluid and is an ideal complement to a detox programme.

### A network of channels

The human body is equipped with another system of channels, in addition to the veins and arteries: those in which the body's 2 litres (4 pints) of lymph circulate. This whitish, milky fluid is the body's refuse collector. It absorbs metabolic waste from around the cells, enters the lymphatic system and then heads towards the collarbone. Around here it enters the vena cava, the body's

### ● ● ● DID YOU KNOW?

> It takes about ten sessions to achieve a significant improvement. For a few hours after each session you feel a strong need to urinate. This indicates that the kidneys are filtering out waste matter more rapidly.

> Lymphatic drainage is thought to help remove those unsightly lumpy accumulations of water, fats and waste we know as cellulite.

main vein, which channels blood to the heart. Now that it's in the bloodstream, the waste matter can be transported to the body's main excretory organs.

One interesting aspect of the lymphatic system is that lymph only moves upwards. It has to combat gravity, but, unlike the bloodstream – which has the heart – lymph has no pump to propel it. It solves this problem by employing a system of valves, like lock gates on a canal, which close behind the lymph fluid once it has passed through.

## Gentle but effective massage

When lymph drains too slowly through the tissues, the results are a gradual accumulation of toxins, oedema and water retention. Lymphatic drainage consists of gentle and precise massage, specially designed to improve the circulation of lymph fluid.

The treatment is carried out in beauty salons or by physiotherapists and lasts for about an hour. The massage is so light and gentle that you might feel it can't be doing any good. But it certainly is! Lymphatic drainage, when well performed, substantially improves the removal of waste matter by accelerating the circulation of the lymph fluid that cleanses the body.

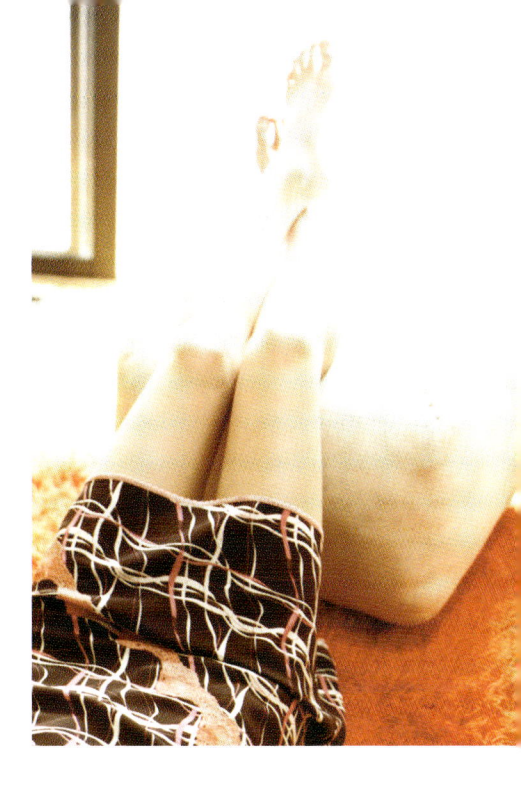

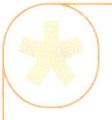

### KEY FACTS

* Lymph fluid circulates upwards through the lymph vessels.

* It collects cellular waste and carries towards excretion.

* Lymphatic drainage improves the circulation of lymph fluid and the elimination of the waste matter it contains.

# 26 massage your feet

**A good foot massage is very relaxing. Of course, if your body is relaxed, it accumulates less waste than when it's stressed. But if you massage the right parts of the foot, you'll turn a moment of pleasure into a genuine detox treatment.**

## The map on your feet

In India and China, for example, massage is a daily feature of a healthy lifestyle. Parents massage their children; the young massage the old. The sole of the foot is a kind of map of our whole body. By massaging the zones corresponding to each bodily organ, we can stimulate its activity. There are other reflex zones besides the feet – for instance, the ears (auriculotherapy), the iris of the eye (iridology) and the hands.

### ● ● ● DID YOU KNOW?

> There are other important points on the sole of the foot.
> Massage the centre of the arch on both feet: they correspond to the kidneys.

> If you then work down to the heel, moving to the outside of the foot, you will stimulate the colon.

There are three parts to a massage session. First, gently massage the whole foot with cream or oil. Next, concentrate on the areas you've selected, beginning with those on the top of the foot and moving to those on the sole. Finally, repeat what you did at the beginning of the session. If a particular point or zone is painful, don't worry. This means you have located an organ that needs some stimulation. Keep massaging it!

## Give your feet a hand

To improve the removal of waste matter, you need to work particularly on the points that correspond to the lymph nodes. On its travels through the body, the lymph fluid leaves some of its load in the nodes. Waste and toxins collect there to be filtered. By stimulating these noses, you can accelerate the excretion of the waste deposited there by the lymph fluid.

The points corresponding to the lymph nodes in the upper body are on the toes, particularly the big toe. Massage them vigorously on top, underneath and at the point where they join the rest of the foot. You also need to massage the ankle area, which corresponds to the lymphatic nodes in the lower half of the body.

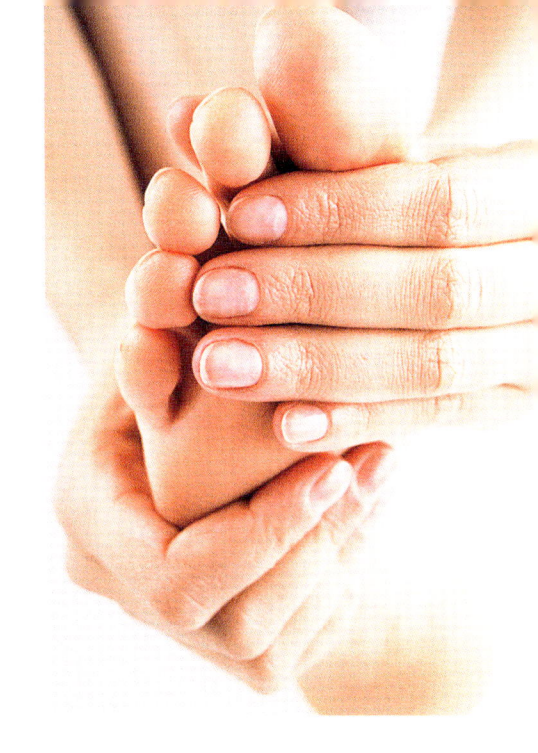

### KEY FACTS

* Foot reflexology stimulates your body's excretory organs by means of massage.

* Concentrate on the toes and the ankle area.

* On the sole of your foot, work on the middle of the arch and then gradually work down to the heel.

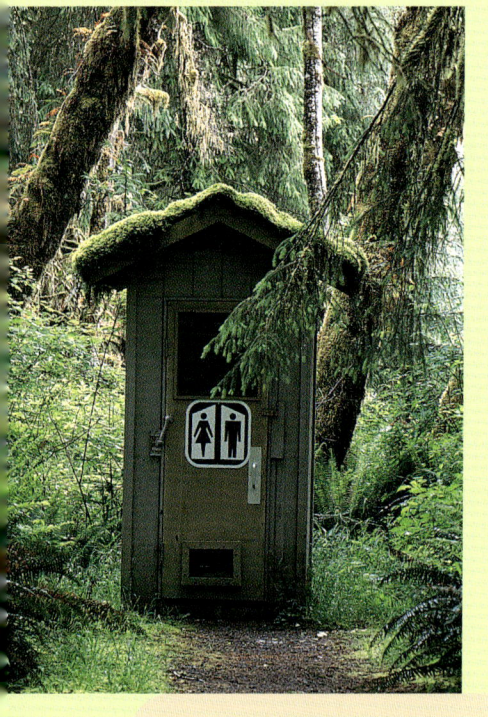

# 27 plants that are good for the kidneys

The kidneys' arduous task never ceases. Day and night, they filter, carry away and eliminate. And they are fantastic at their job, but they can still benefit from a little help. Java tea (orthosiphon), mouse-ear hawkweed and cherry stalks all offer that help.

### ••• DID YOU KNOW?

> Herbal tea made from cherry stalks is another gentle diuretic that's been used since time immemorial.

> In his *Natural History*, Pliny the Elder relates that a cherry tree was brought back to Rome by Lucullus after his victory over Mithridates. So we owe Lucullus a double debt of gratitude, for the tree's delicious, purifying fruit as well as for its stalks.

## A little flower from Java

Orthosiphon grows in wet, hot regions such as Java, India, Australia, and Malaysia, where it is called 'cat's whisker' because of its wispy stamens. It is dried and drunk as tea. The plant is best known for its amazing diuretic qualities. It rapidly increases urine volume and accelerates its excretion. However, unlike artificial diuretic drugs, Java tea acts only while there are toxins and excess water in the body. This quality means that it never causes dehydration.

Java tea is available in capsules. A course would normally be four to six capsules each day for a month. Alternatively, it can be consumed in the traditional way, as herbal tea. Put 2 tablespoonfuls into 500ml (1 pint) of boiling water and infuse for 10 minutes. Some care needs to be taken with this product, though – do not use it if you have any heart or kidney problems and always consume plenty of fluid during the day.

## Small, but very effective

Mouse-ear hawkweed is a small, flowery plant that particularly helps remove excess urea from the body. It has been used in traditional folk medicine to treat heart and kidney problems, oedema and uraemia. It certainly increases urine flow! In days gone by the plant was soaked in white wine and taken at the rate of 2 or 3 tablespoonfuls a day. It's now available in capsule form and as a herbal tea. Put 25g (1oz) of hawkweed in 500ml (1 pint) of boiling water and infuse for 10 minutes. Up to three cups a day should be fine, but be careful when using this plant – if you suffer from heart or kidney problems, consult a doctor before taking it.

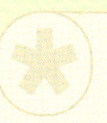

### KEY FACTS

* Plants are excellent aids for your kidneys.

* Java tea and mouse-ear hawkweed are powerful diuretics that are safer than diuretic drugs. They can be consumed as herbal teas or in capsule form.

* Herbal tea made from cherry stalks is also very effective.

> To make herbal tea out of the latter, put a tablespoonful of dried stalks in a large cup of cold water. Boil the mixture for five minutes, allow to cool until lukewarm, then strain before drinking.

# 28 poultices will do the trick

Different poultices have been used for centuries to treat a huge variety of illnesses. When correctly applied, clay and cabbage poultices stimulate the excretory organs.

### It's a kind of plaster

The procedure for making a plant poultice is straightforward. You take as much of the plant as you need (it varies from plant to plant), boil it for between two and twenty minutes (again, it varies), then drain it carefully. (Don't let the decoction go to waste: it can be used as either a herbal tea or a lotion.) Leave the

● ● ● DID YOU KNOW?

> Clay poultices also help the excretory organs to do their work. Add pure, lukewarm water to powdered clay to make a thick paste. Stir until all the lumps have been removed and then spread the paste on to a fine cloth.

> Place the cloth on the area over your liver, lungs or kidneys and keep it there for about twenty minutes. These poultices cleanse and stimulate the organs concerned.

boiled plant to cool for about ten minutes. In the meantime, put a little sweet almond oil on your skin above the organ to be treated: for example, on the lower back if you want to drain and stimulate your kidneys; just below and to the right of the rib cage if you are treating your liver. When the plants have cooled down sufficiently to be applied comfortably, place them on the appropriate spot and cover them with a fine, clean cloth. Leave the poultice in place for at least half an hour.

## Large green leaves

The cabbage is undoubtedly the most effective plant to use in a poultice for the kidneys. Before going to bed, remove the thickest veins from the leaves of a cabbage and then boil what's left for two minutes. When it has cooled, spread the poultice on the skin and leave it there all night. Cabbage is powerfully absorbent, so the poultice extracts waste from the body's tissues. It's also very rich in mineral salts, so it nourishes the body while cleansing it. Milan cabbage makes the best poultice but other varieties work well, too.

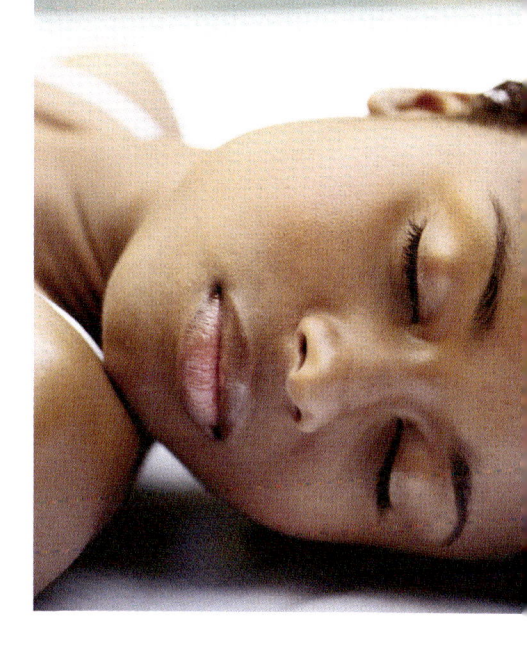

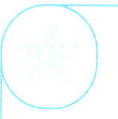

### KEY FACTS

* Poultices are very easy to make: boil the plant and apply it to the skin.

* Cabbage has a strong cleansing effect and also supplies the body with minerals.

* Clay also thoroughly cleans the excretory organs.

# 29 eat plenty of charcoal

**Eating charcoal may seem an odd idea but it is an old remedy that has stood the test of time. Like clay, charcoal has properties that cleanse the body.**

**All the purity of carbon** Charcoal is produced when certain kinds of wood - – such as willow, lime and poplar – are burnt. It is pure carbon, but when the wood is burnt at a high temperature and steamed, it becomes riddled with tiny cavities. The charcoal can then be formed into a pastille, which, when swallowed, traps any organic waste it encounters.

**Additives, pollutants and germs** The pastille is not broken down by digestive juices, so it remains intact during its passage through the body. Along the way, the remnants of drugs, metabolic waste, food additives, pollutants and other undesirable substances become trapped in the carbon and are then excreted along with it. Charcoal is even able to eliminate intestinal germs, and, when in the intestines, attracts, holds and carries away toxins in the blood.

### DID YOU KNOW?

> Charcoal is available in the following forms: powder, granules, capsules and pastilles. Each form has its own advantages and disadvantages. The capsules, for example, contain only a small amount of charcoal but they have no unpleasant taste, which can be a problem for some people.

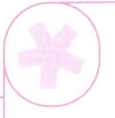

### KEY FACTS

* Charcoal attracts toxins that are present in the digestive system and eliminates them through the intestines.

* Charcoal is readily available in various forms.

# 30 buy a hot-water bottle

Yet another remedy that has been used for centuries is the humble hot-water bottle. Our grandmothers knew all about its beneficial properties and we should as well.

**The amazing liver!** Warmth helps the liver to function, and a simple way to achieve this is to place a heat source directly over the top of it. The liver works incessantly to eliminate harmful substances. It destroys germs and viruses, and neutralizes toxic chemicals, such as food additives and drugs, that could have dangerous side-effects. Blood that is full of dead cells and excess cholesterol is pumped through it and cleansed. The extra boost of heat supplied by a hot-water bottle is though to help it to combat colic caused by gall stones.

**Treat your liver well...** The liver secretes a substance called bile, which is collected by the bile ducts and stored in the gall bladder When you eat, hormones cause the gall bladder to contract and send bile into the gut to help with the absorption of fat.

### ● ● ● DID YOU KNOW?

> Bile is a mixture of salts, cholesterol and bilirubin (the breakdown product of red cells). If its composition changes, cholesterol crystals begin to form in the gall bladder and make gall stones. These might have no ill-effects, but could lead to severe pain or even jaundice. So it pays to treat your liver well.

### KEY FACTS

* The liver performs a wide variety of cleansing functions.

* Bile, essential for digestion, is produced by the liver.

* Placing a hot-water bottle over the liver can help it to function.

# 31
## the olive: a tree of many talents

**Olives are a treat for the eyes in the Mediterranean countryside and a treat for the taste buds because of their sweet-smelling, delicious oil. The olive is also a genuinely medicinal plant, with both its leaves and its fruit possessing therapeutic qualities.**

### First the leaves…

Olive leaf extract combats a number of viruses, bacteria and fungi. This is largely due to the oleuropein contained within it. Of course, taking the extract doesn't guarantee a lifetime free from illness, but it forms an important part of a detox programme, because it flushes numerous dormant germs out of the system. Take 2g ($^1/_{15}$oz) of the extract each day.

### ●●● DID YOU KNOW?

> A diet rich in olive oil may well keep you healthy and let you enjoy a long life, which is hardly surprising as olive trees themselves are famously long-lived. Some of the tress still thriving today on the Mount of Olives in Jerusalem were there when Jesus was a visitor.

> Although they originated in Asia Minor and the Mediterranean, olives are now cultivated all over the world, and their health benefits are recognized as far afield as Japan and South America.

Olive leaf tea is less effective against germs but nevertheless can make a useful component of a detox treatment: it dilates the arteries and improves blood circulation, which, in turn, helps the excretory organs to perform their duties. It has slight diuretic qualities and, in particular, helps to eliminate urea. It also cleanses the liver and the gall bladder. To make the tea, use 1 tablespoonful of chopped leaves per large cup of cold water, boil for three minutes and then strain. Ideally, drink it in the morning before eating.

### … then the oil

As part of a Mediterranean diet rich in fruit, vegetables and complex carbohydrates, olive oil appears to protect against both coronary artery disease and cancer of the colon. The beneficial health effects of olive oil are due to both its high content of monounsaturated fatty acids and its high content of antioxidative substances. It is also very well tolerated by the stomach, and its protective function has a beneficial effect on gastritis and ulcers. So use olive oil, preferably extra virgin and organic, in cooking and for salad dressings.

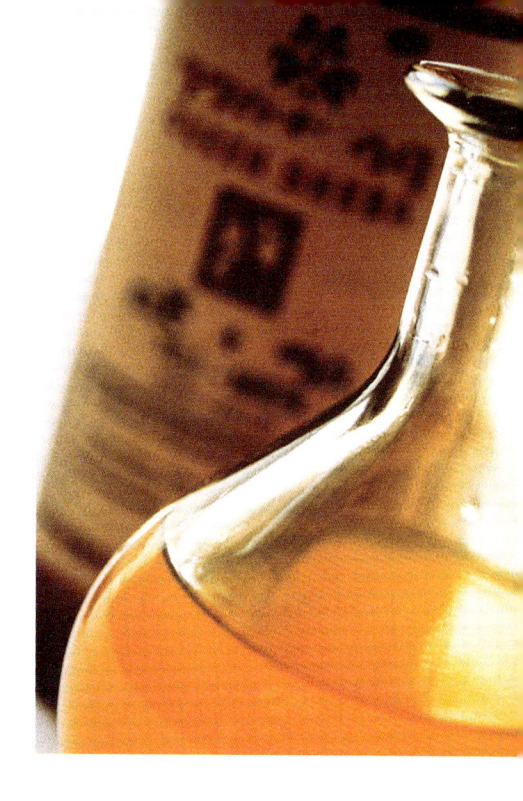

### KEY FACTS

* Olive leaf extract helps to eliminate fungi, bacteria and viruses from the body.

* Olive leaf tea is cleansing and is a diuretic.

* Olive oil is believed to protect against both heart disease and cancer.

# 32 plants that are good for the liver

Because of its many functions, the liver is particularly susceptible to toxic overload, and sometimes it needs quite vigorous help. Fortunately, there are certain medicinal plants, such as boldo, lime-tree sapwood, milk thistle and peppermint, that are guaranteed to help.

## Help the body's reprocessing plant

Besides purifying the blood, the liver has other functions: for instance, it stores vitamins and glucose, and it metabolizes hormones. It's hardly surprising, then, that the liver is sometimes overworked. Boldo has a tonic effect on the liver and stimulates the secretion of bile. Use it when you've had too much to eat or drink. A word of warning, though: boldo should not be used to attempt to treat

### ●●● DID YOU KNOW?

> Thyme and rosemary add wonderful flavours to food, but these aromatic herbs also do wonders for a sluggish liver. Rosemary, especially, is strongly choleretic; that is, it increases bile secretion.

> You can also drink it as a herbal tea (it's delicious!) in the evening, after dinner. Put a teaspoonful of rosemary in a cup of boiling water and let it infuse for ten minutes.

serious cases of liver damage. To make a herbal tea, use 10g (1/3oz) of boldo per litre (2 pints) of boiling water and leave to infuse for 10 minutes. Drink a cup before each meal.

Peppermint stimulates and cleanses the gall bladder. Put a teaspoonful of the plant into a cup of boiling water and leave to infuse for ten minutes. Drink a cup after meals.

## More helpful plants

Thanks to its high flavonoid content, lime-tree sapwood stimulates sluggish livers. It also helps to relieve headaches caused by liver disorders, as well as feelings of nausea. To make a decoction, use a tablespoonful of sapwood per cup of cold water and boil for three minutes. Drink three cups each day, sweetened with honey if desired.

Milk thistle has excellent draining qualities because of the presence in the plant of silymarin, a substance that protects liver cells. A short period of treatment with milk thistle will help you to recover from a bout of overeating. To make a herbal tea, use a tablespoonful of the plant per 250ml (1/2 pint) of boiling water. Drink a cup before meals for a fortnight to help your digestive system to recover.

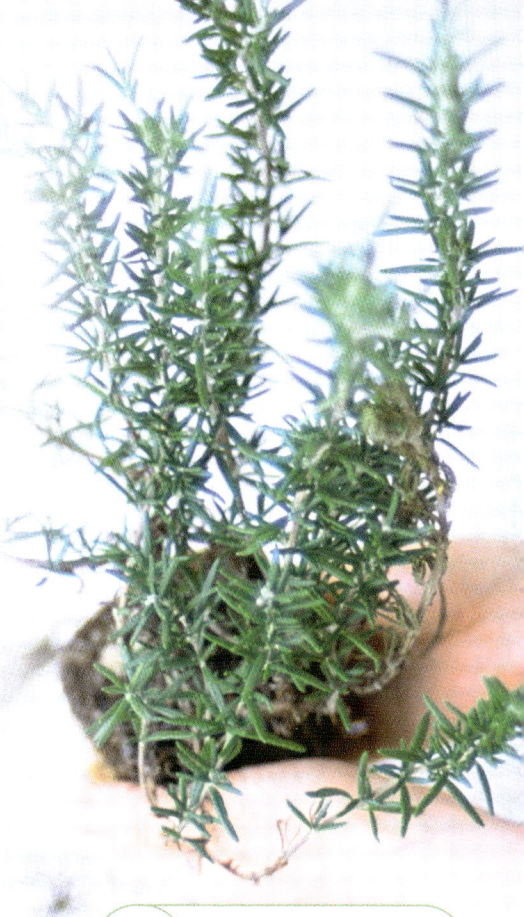

### KEY FACTS

* To help your liver in a more vigorous way, try plants like lime-tree sapwood, milk thistle, peppermint and boldo.

* Don't forget to use thyme and rosemary when cooking.

# 33 beating constipation

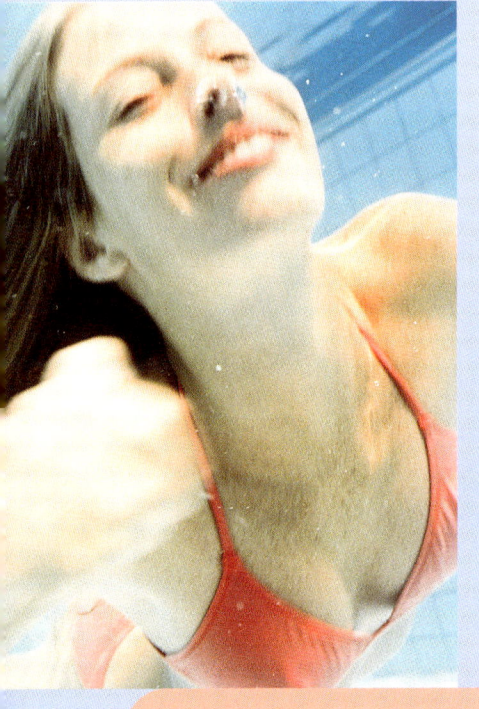

Many people suffer from constipation at some time or another. It causes abdominal pain, wind and bloating, aggravates haemorrhoids, and can cause painful tears (anal fissures) around the anus if the stools are very hard. In other words, it's much more serious than you might think, and it must be cured.

### DID YOU KNOW?

> Flax seeds are rich in fibre and polyunsaturated fatty acids, which means they are a gentle but effective laxative.

> They also contain mucilage, which, when mixed with water, produces a gel that increases stool volume. They also soothe bowels made 'irritable' by chronic constipation.

## Beware of the side-effects of drugs

An unhealthy complexion, bloated stomach and rings around the eyes are all signs of chronic constipation. It's hardly surprising that there's so much of it about. Many of the evils of the Western world – lack of exercise, high levels of stress, low-fibre diets – cause the intestines to become sluggish, indeed almost dormant. The overuse of tranquillizers does nothing to help, either. Laxative medicines may work in the short term but are not a long-term solution. Initially they speed up excretion, but if you continue to take them, they eventually have the opposite effect: the intestines come to rely on them and become more sluggish than ever.

## Water, exercise and regularity

Instead, it's better to abide by the rules of a healthy lifestyle: eat enough dietary fibre (see Tip 18); help the alimentary canal to do its work by thoroughly chewing each mouthful of food; drink plenty of water; and take exercise. This final point is often overlooked, but strong abdominal muscles are essential if the bowels are to function properly. To help develop these muscles, take regular gentle exercise, such as walking or swimming. Regular use of these important muscles improves muscle contraction within the intestines, which is vital to good excretion.

In addition, try to retrain your bowels by passing motions at regular times and, crucially, going whenever you feel the need. The best time for most people is in the morning after breakfast.

> You can eat raw flax seeds, provided you chew them well, or drink them in a herbal tea. Put 50g (2oz) in 1 litre (2 pints) of boiling water and leave them to infuse for at least 2 hours. Drink the liquid sweetened with honey.

### KEY FACTS

* Constipation causes abdominal pain and bloating

* To cure the problem, abide by the rules a healthy lifestyle: take exercise, drink plenty of water, eat fibre.

* Flax seeds are a useful natural laxative.

# 34 plants that are good for the intestines

Each year, millions of laxatives are sold to (often embarrassed) customers in pharmacies. But the embarrassment, and some more important side-effects, can be avoided by looking to nature for a solution. Plant remedies are gentler than chemical laxatives, last longer and don't irritate the bowels.

## Nature's best laxative

Alder buckthorn is often considered top of the bill when it comes to curing constipation. Its biggest virtue is that it doesn't irritate the bowels. However, don't take too much of it at first, and increase the dosage gradually, because alder buckthorn is potent. It also stimulates bile secretion. Use ¹/₂ teaspoonful of the plant per 250ml (¹/₂ pint) of cold

### ●●● DID YOU KNOW?

> The husk of the ispaghula seed is very rich in mucilage. When it comes into contact with water in the digestive tract, it forms a gel. This cannot be absorbed by the body, so it increases the volume of stools. (The effect is very similar to that produced by flax seeds – see Tip 33.)

> The gel also carries bile salts away to excretion, so forcing the liver to produce a new batch. This is highly beneficial because bile salts are made from cholesterol; when the liver is forced to make more, it has to extract cholesterol from the blood.

water, boil for 5 minutes, then remove from the heat and leave to infuse for a further 10 minutes. Sweeten with honey and drink a cup before going to bed.

## Mallow and marsh mallow

Pythagoras once said of mallow, 'It is suitable for calming the passions and keeping the stomach and the spirit free.' Nowadays it is known to be a plant with harmless laxative properties that can even sooth inflamed intestines. Put a tablespoonful of the plant in a cup of boiling water and allow it to infuse for ten minutes.

Marsh mallow also has similar soothing effects on irritated intestines. Use 15g ($^1/_2$ oz) of the leaves for every 500ml (1 pint) of water, leave to infuse for 10 minutes, sweeten with honey and drink 3 cups a day.

> Ispaghula is sold in pharmacies in sachet and capsule forms. It should always be taken with plenty of water. To avoid wind, increase the dose gradually, and take advice from your doctor if you have any gut problems.

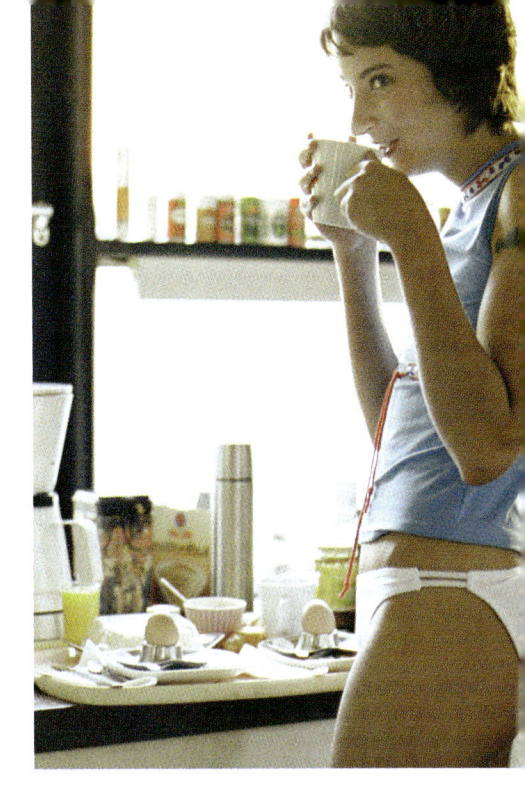

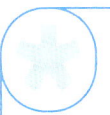

### KEY FACTS

* Some plants have laxative properties and can relieve constipation.

* Plants cause much less bowel irritation and inflammation than commercial laxatives.

* Try mallow, marsh mallow, alder buckthorn and ispaghula.

# 35 consider colonic irrigation

**In the past, enemas were commonplace. Today, some doctors advise colonic irrigation, although others are sceptical about its benefits. It should always be considered carefully.**

**Water and a pump…** Enemas were widely used until the 1950s in the treatment of constipation. The technique is simple: lukewarm water is injected into the rectum by means of a pump. The pump is then withdrawn and the contents of the intestines pass out of the body in the customary way. This basic method is used much less today.

**Filtered, salty water** Some exponents of natural medicine have made colonic irrigation, or colonic hydrotherapy, popular. The principle is similar to that of an enema: the patient lies down and a machine introduces filtered, usually salty, water into the colon and then flushes it out again. Three sessions are required for the method to make a real difference. According to its supporters, colonic irrigation is a thorough and effective method of eliminating a build-up of intestinal toxins.

### ● ● ● DID YOU KNOW?

> Colonic irrigation is advocated as a way of cleansing the body and treating constipation, diarrhoea, colitis and some autoimmune illnesses. The procedure should be avoided if you are pregnant, extremely tired or suffering from serious illnesses of the colon.

### KEY FACTS

* In the past, intestinal enemas were often used.

* Nowadays, some doctors advocate colonic irrigation.

* It is a controversial technique that must not be performed under certain circumstances.

# 36 have a really good laugh

**What cure could be more enjoyable than a good fit of the giggles? Laughter is beneficial for respiration, blood circulation and the secretion of hormones.**

**A good clean out** When we have a good laugh, the whole body gets cleaned out. Our normal rhythm of breathing is broken and our lungs are jerkily, but thoroughly, emptied before filling up again. These jolting movements of the diaphragm massage the abdominal cavity, so that all its organs, particularly the intestines, are stimulated. What's more, heart rate and blood circulation are accelerated, which improves the expulsion of waste matter from the blood.

**The happiness hormones** Laughter also stimulates the secretion of certain hormones in the brain. The level of endorphins shows a marked rise, bringing mental relaxation and a mild sense of euphoria. As a result, you laugh even more. When you are less stressed and tense, your whole body relaxes: everything functions better, including the elimination of waste matter.

### DID YOU KNOW?

> In Western societies we're losing the habit of laughing. Research suggests that a hundred years ago we laughed for twenty minutes a day. We're now down to five minutes. It's high time laughter was brought back into fashion. Friends could organize theme parties with the sole aim of making everyone laugh.

### KEY FACTS

* Laughter changes the breathing pattern, so the abdominal cavity is massaged.

* Heart rate and blood circulation speed up, causing more waste to be filtered from the blood.

* The body functions better and eliminates waste more efficiently.

# 37 massage your stomach

Jin shin do (*do-in*) is a massage technique that forms part of traditional Chinese medicine. It is founded on the same principles as acupuncture: life-giving vital energy can be stimulated by acting upon specific points on the body. In jin shin do, however, you use your fingers, not needles.

## The points of balance and harmony

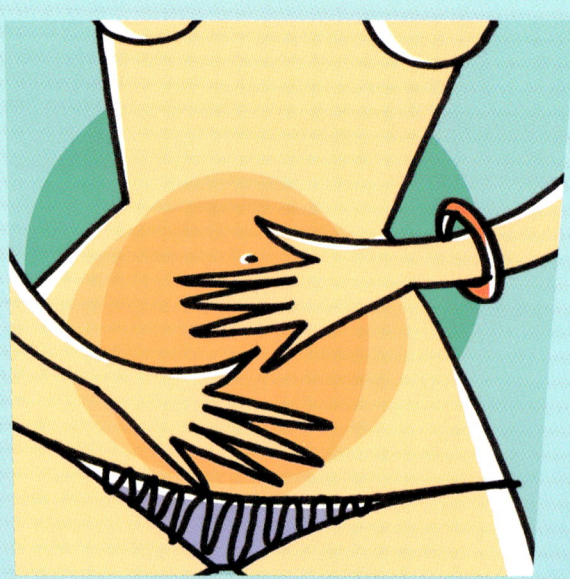

In Chinese medicine, health is all a matter of harmony: between the world and ourselves, and, above all, between the different energy meridians within us. These meridians are like channels in which the vital fluid, or energy, circulates, feeding the organs, balancing bodily functions and maintaining life. When the smooth flow of energy is disrupted, so there is too much blocked in one place and not enough elsewhere, illnesses occur.

This applies to the excretory organs as much as to all the others. The condition of the liver, kidneys, intestines and skin, for example, is governed by this energy. To ensure that a proper balance is maintained, specific points along the energy meridians need to be stimulated. This is done by pressing hard on each point and massaging it firmly with the inside of the fingers, turning first in one direction, then the other.

## How to massage the liver and intestines

The points that stimulate the intestines are on the stomach. With your finger, trace a line from the solar plexus down through the navel to the pubic area. Then trace two parallel lines a hand's width to the right and the left of the middle line. These are the two lines you need to massage, moving upwards from the bottom of each line. Some of the points will be more sensitive than others, and you should concentrate on these.

The points that stimulate the liver are a little higher up, on the chest. First, draw your fingers across the bottom of your ribs. Work particularly on any painful points that you find. Then, trace a line across your chest on a level with your nipples. Massage along this line, concentrating on the sensitive points.

### ●●● DID YOU KNOW?

> If a point is painful to the touch, then you've located a blocked energy point.

> Initially, you should not apply too much pressure on the point: you don't want the pain to become unbearable.

> As soon as you feel the pain and the blockage starting to ease, you can start to press a little harder.

### KEY FACTS

* Jin shin do is a massage technique used in traditional Chinese medicine.

* You press with the inside of your fingers the points on the body that correspond to the organs you want to stimulate.

* Those points corresponding to the intestines are on the stomach and those corresponding to the liver are on the chest.

## 38 take a deep breath

**The lungs excrete waste material every time we exhale. To help them perform this vital function, and clean their billions of tiny air sacs, take a deep breath!**

### We breathe badly!

The lungs are like sponges. Billions of tiny alveoli (air sacs) absorb the air we breathe and filter it. Oxygen passes into the blood through their thin walls, while, in return, the alveoli receive waste gases, mainly carbon dioxide, from the blood. These waste gases are expelled when we exhale. However, because we usually breathe too shallowly, sometimes in polluted atmospheres, our lungs have difficulty expelling all the waste.

### DID YOU KNOW?

> Learn to improve your breathing. We tend never to fill or empty our lungs completely.
> As often as you can, spend a few moments breathing deeply: inhale until your lungs are completely full and hold your breath for three seconds; then slowly exhale until your lungs are completely empty, pushing with your abdominal muscles to ensure that all the air has been expelled; keep your lungs empty for three seconds and then repeat.

## Dry or wet inhalation?

There's nothing better for cleaning the alveoli than inhaling plant essential oils. When we breathe them in deeply, their active particles penetrate into the deep recesses of the lungs.

**Dry inhalation:** put some drops of a carefully chosen essential oil (see Tip 39) either on your pillow before you go to bed or on a cotton handkerchief, so that you can inhale it several times during the day.

**Wet inhalation:** pour ten drops of essential oil into a bowl of steaming water. Cover your head with a towel and bend your head over the bowl. Inhale the steam for five minutes.

> Concentrate on the long, slow breath out. This will calm you and help you avoid overbreathing (hyperventilating).

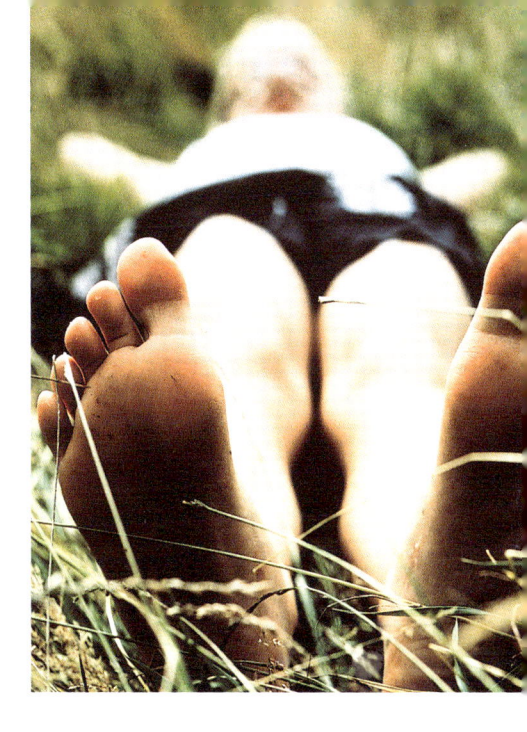

### KEY FACTS

* The lungs expel waste matter in the air we breathe.

* Their alveoli provide the blood with oxygen in exchange for carbon dioxide.

* To help your lungs, try using wet or dry inhalations.

* Train yourself to breathe deeply..

# 39 plants that are good for breathing

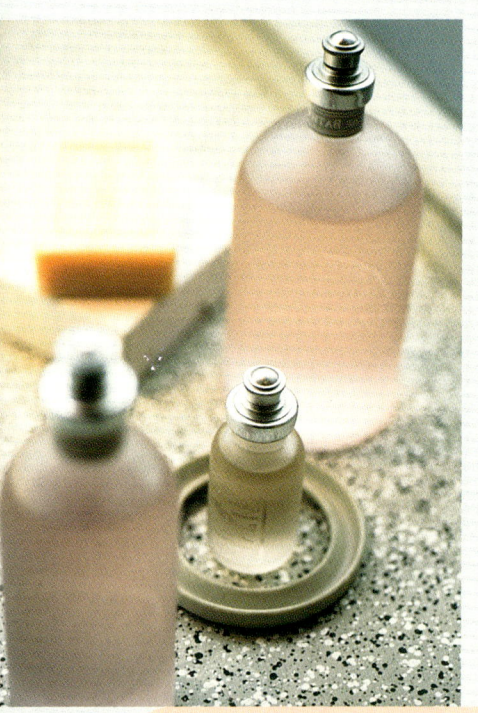

Particular plants are effective when used in inhalations. Eucalyptus thyme, lavender and pine all have the capacity to give your lungs a thorough cleansing. And they smell great too!

### DID YOU KNOW?

> You can make up your mixture of essential oils in advance and keep it in an airtight bottle.

> Make sure that the bottle is not transparent because light can damage the active principles. Store in a cool, dry place.

## First and foremost, eucalyptus

The leaves and young branches of the eucalyptus tree produce a free-flowing essential oil with a pungent but pleasant fragrance. When you inhale it you are smelling the eucalyptol. This is such an active ingredient that eucalyptus trees are even known to have a purifying effect on the atmosphere surrounding them.

Eucalyptol has a powerful antiseptic quality that helps to destroy germs in the lungs, whether they are active or dormant. It also contributes to the removal of mucus, which often congests the respiratory tract.

There are more than seven hundred different varieties of eucalyptus trees, but all contain enough eucalyptol to kill germs in the respiratory tract effectively. To improve the effectiveness of your inhalations, mix eucalyptus with other plant oils.

> You can vary the proportions of the oils according to your symptoms (dry cough, loose cough, irritation, etc.) and to how fragrant you find them.

## Try mixing these essential oils with your eucalyptus

**Thyme:** contains the powerful antiseptic thymol. It is also anti-inflammatory and therefore suitable for treating lungs that have been congested for a long time and become inflamed.

**Lavender:** as well as killing germs, lavender has antispasmodic and sedative qualities. It can soothe inflamed bronchial tubes and alleviate ticklish coughs. Some varieties are better than others: try to find *Lavandula angustifolia* or *Lavandula officinalis*.

**Pine:** stimulates our immune system and helps the body to eliminate harmful waste.

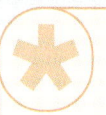

### KEY FACTS

* Eucalyptus should be your first choice of essential oil to use as an inhalation.

* You can mix it with pine, lavender or thyme.

* Mix the oils according to your symptoms and to achieve the most pleasant scent.

# 40 take your time

**A detox programme needs to be prepared and followed carefully and sensibly. Don't expect to cleanse your body of all its toxins in three days.**

**Slowly but surely** Although some treatments and monodiets only last a few days, they must be components of a much longer programme if they are to succeed. If you really want to rid your body of all its toxins, you must be prepared to undergo a three- to four-week detox, which will have to be repeated two, three or even four times each year.

**Preparation is the key** The first time you try a detox treatment, pay particular attention to the build-up. Plan to take several weeks over this and don't rush through the different dietary changes. Give your excretory organs all the help you can by using plants, essential oils and massage. Subsequently, you may gradually shorten the preparatory stage and try tougher monodiets, and even a course of fasting.

### DID YOU KNOW?

> Keep a record of all your sensations and symptoms in order to improve future detox programmes. Certain reactions, such as spots and halitosis, could occur during the programme. These are the outward signs of the different stages of the internal cleansing.

### KEY FACTS

* Don't kid yourself: in three days you're not going to eliminate all the waste that has been accumulating for years. Take your time!

* The first time you detox, concentrate on the preparatory phase.

# case study

**My liver was overloaded with toxins and I didn't know!**

« For years, I regularly suffered from spots on my face that would not budge. I felt tired, and during the winter I always caught colds and flu. What's more, my digestion was very slow, and I used to fall asleep after meals. But I never put two and two together. One day I read an article in a magazine about a detox programme. I liked the idea and decided to try it, but it was terrible: I got twice as many spots as before and felt more tired than ever. So I went to see a medical herbalist, who explained that my liver had been overloaded with toxins for years and was merely going through the process of being cleaned. That had been the cause of all my troubles! He advised me to drink herbal teas and follow a strict diet. And after a few weeks I was feeling good: no spots, no tiredness. Now I follow a little detox programme at the beginning of each new season and everything's fine. »

# 41 >>>

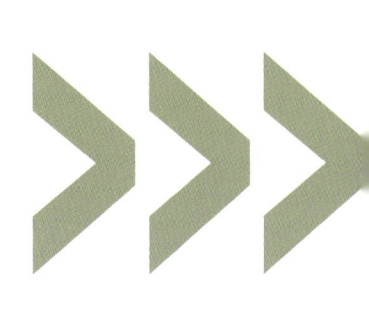

>> We are not only polluted by toxic chemicals and food additives. **Bad habits, anger, stress, fear, anxiety and obsessive behaviour** are all harmful to our health.

>>>> Unfortunately, there are no excretory organs to eliminate these things. We have to rely on our brains and nervous systems, and they can't just flush them out of us. **We have to be consciously determined to do something about them.**

>>>>>> This is not something that can be achieved overnight, but it's certainly possible. **Then, with the body cleansed and the heart light**, you will finally feel your true self again!

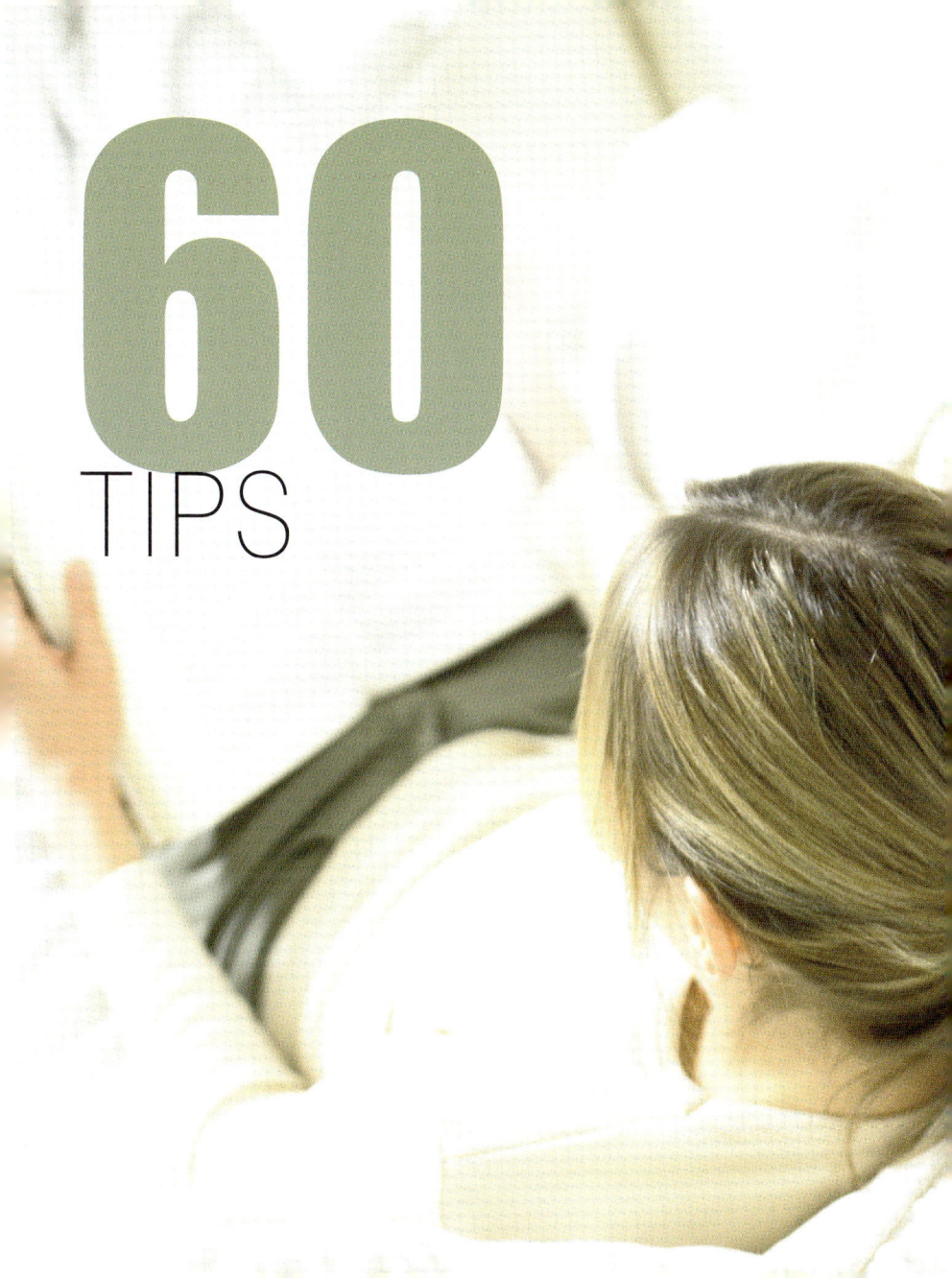

# 60 TIPS

# 41
## come to terms with stress

It's a word on everyone's lips and makes headlines in all the magazines. Stress is blamed for everything. However, although it can obviously be harmful, it's possible to turn it to our advantage, provided we understand it.

### Can stress be good for you?

Stress, in itself, is neither good nor bad. But it stimulates us, makes us react, take action, run away or fight. Without it, early humans never would have adapted to their environment, never would have developed and evolved, never would have survived. Without stress, we would not be here! However, this indispensable stimulation can also work against us. When stressful circumstances become

### DID YOU KNOW?

> Meditation, relaxation, making time to enjoy yourself, sports and creative activities are all effective ways to cope with too much stress and keep difficult problems at a distance. On the other hand, they can all also be tailored to ensure that you still benefit from the positive aspects of stress.

> Some plants, such as marjoram, ginseng and St John's wort, are very good for helping us to adapt to stressful circumstances. St John's wort should not be taken in conjunction with anti-depressants.

too painful or too violent, when they occur too frequently and we have no defence against them, they gradually damage us. Our minds feel the strain first: we become confused, unable to cope and emotionally hypersensitive. Then the body starts to suffer too. When we are overstressed, a storm of hormonal activity disrupts the body's normal functioning and ever more toxins accumulate inside us.

## A response system that's lost its value

Humans know how to respond to stress. We do it automatically. When we experience a violent emotion, our heart rate accelerates to pump more blood to the parts of the body that need it: the muscles, so we can either run away or stay and fight; and the brain, so we can think fast on our feet. A surge of adrenaline floods into the bloodstream to help the body mobilize its resources. Nowadays, however, we live in a society where neither fighting nor running away is usually the most appropriate reaction. All the body's highly tuned rapid responses have been for nothing! Eventually, all this pointless internal effort takes its toll. Therefore, combating or, better still, coming to terms with stress needs to be a key part of a thorough detox programme.

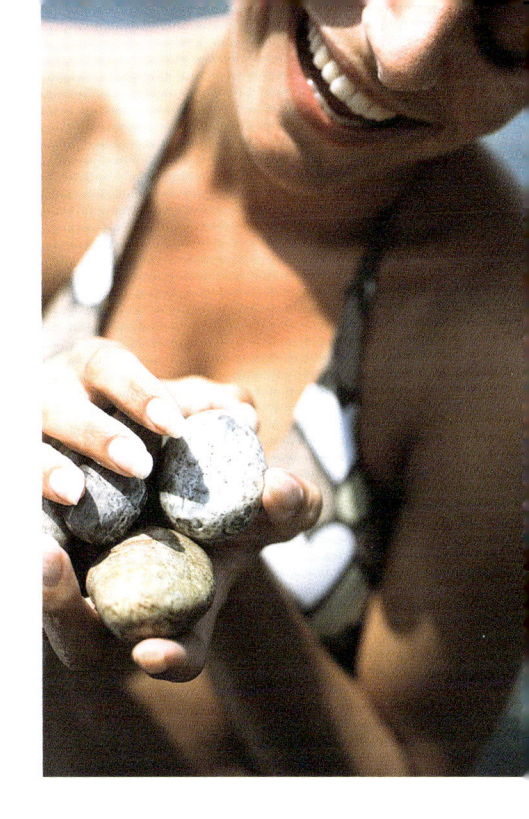

### KEY FACTS

* Stress itself is neither good nor bad.

* Excess stress gradually wears us down.

* To come to terms with stress, you need to relax, enjoy yourself and exercise.

# 42
## learn to relax

Relaxation is without doubt the best way to deal with stress. The word covers myriad techniques, some of which date back millennia, although their image has changed greatly over the last thirty years. Their essential principles remain the same as ever: breathing and concentration.

### Anxiety and its physical symptoms

The body and mind are inextricably linked, and this is particularly true when we experience stress and tension. Many different muscles tighten when the mind starts to race, and our breathing becomes tense when we're feeling low. It's as if anxiety and all its physical symptoms are able to capitalize on the slightest psychological or physical crack

● ● ● DID YOU KNOW?

> The spiritual aspect is more important in meditation. Every religion has its form of meditation: Christianity and Islam have prayer, Zen has its poses and Hindu its yoga.

> The practitioners of these methods empty their minds in order to reach a higher spiritual plane. Whatever your own objective, this procedure creates a mood of deep calm.

and worm their way inside to subtly wear us down.

Stress is not a modern-day creation, although the way we live today does seem to welcome it with open arms. For many centuries, and in all civilizations, people have developed techniques to enable them to concentrate and take refuge inside themselves, away from the trials and tribulations of the world. When we start to breathe deeply and rhythmically, our dark thoughts melt away; when our muscles relax, our minds begin to calm.

## Sophrology, autogenic training, meditation

Breathing is at the heart of all these practices: by controlling your breathing, concentrating your mind on this simple, vital rhythm, you distance yourself from the outside world. Other techniques, such as the Jacobson method of relaxation, put the emphasis on consciously relaxing the muscles in order to create a mood of serenity.

Sophrology seeks to change consciousness: a state between wakefulness and sleep is induced, during which you experience relaxing mental images. Autogenic training uses physical sensations, such as heat and the heaviness of the limbs, to produce relaxation. Therapists usually teach you techniques that you can then perform every day by yourself. They all help you gradually to rid yourself of tension and the irritation, annoyance and other negative emotions that it causes.

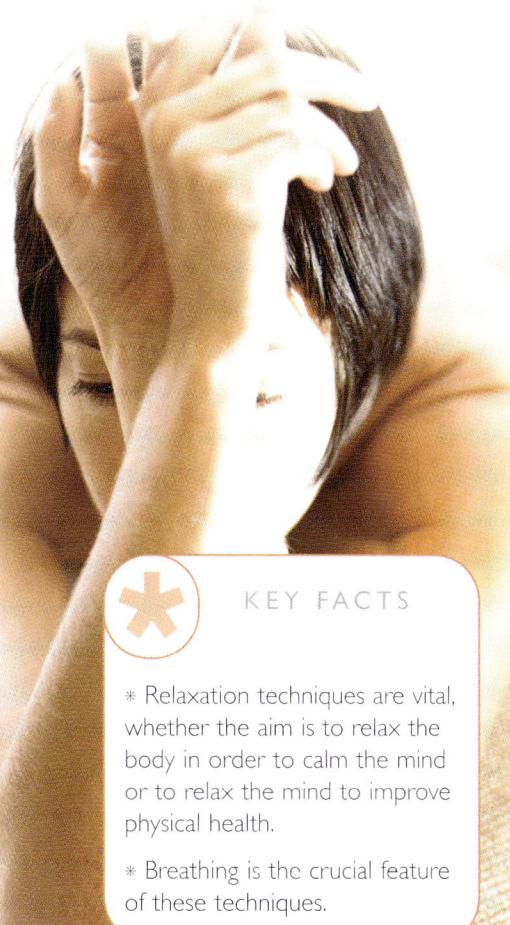

### KEY FACTS

* Relaxation techniques are vital, whether the aim is to relax the body in order to calm the mind or to relax the mind to improve physical health.

* Breathing is the crucial feature of these techniques.

# 43 little bottles of floral essence

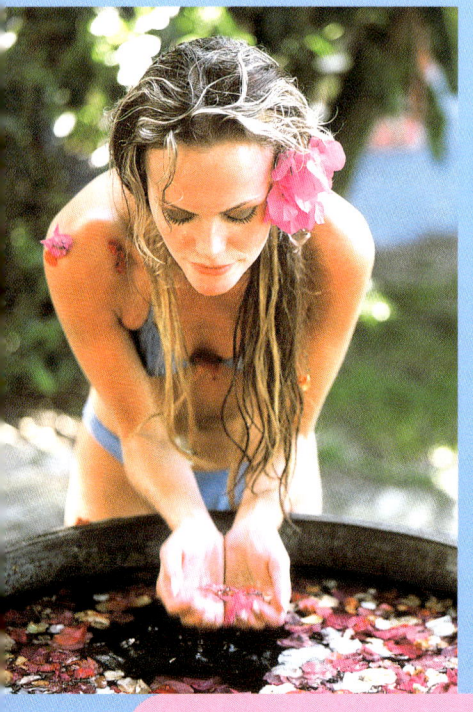

Nature has provided us with many remedies, including flowers. Not only are they beautiful, fragrant and colourful, but they can also help regulate our moods and feelings in the form of floral elixirs.

### DID YOU KNOW?

> Flower elixir concentrates are available from health-food shops and specialist pharmacies.

> You prepare your doses for the day by putting a few drops of the elixir in half a glass of pure water. Drink this over the course of the day, taking a teaspoonful at a time.

## Dr Bach

In the morning flowers open their petals in response to the first rays of the sun. Droplets of dew form on the petals and lie there until it evaporates. It was while watching this timeless process that Dr Edward Bach, an English doctor who lived at the beginning of the 20th century, had the idea of collecting dew from flowers to make an elixir.

Being a good homeopathic doctor (see Tip 46), he saw this process as a natural form of homeopathic dilution. He tested it on some of his patients and was amazed by the results. Above all, the elixirs have an effect our emotions, restoring their balance and regulating their excesses.

Bach set out to achieve two aims: to discover the therapeutic effect of each flower and to develop an easy method of production as close as possible to the original, natural phenomenon. He created thirty-eight different flower elixirs. They are still used throughout the world today.

## Relevant questions and honest answers

Further research has led to the development of new elixirs made from flowers that grow in other parts of the world, such as California, Australia and the Alps. To choose the right elixir, you need to ask yourself relevant questions. For example, how do I feel in the morning when I wake up: anxious, fearful, tense, exhausted? Does this feeling last a long time or disappear rapidly? What change do I hope to achieve? Answer these questions honestly and you'll be able to find the best elixir to help you overcome your difficulties.

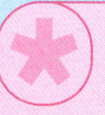

### KEY FACTS

* Floral elixirs were developed by Dr Edward Bach in the first half of the 20th century.

* They help regulate moods and emotions.

* To choose the correct elixir, you must ask yourself relevant questions and answer them honestly.

> You can also put ten or so drops of the elixir in your bathwater.

# 44 elixirs to quell your fears

**If your life is blighted by fear, if panic grips you as soon as you wake up, if there's some ordeal or situation that you dread, try an elixir of aspen or nutmeg.**

**Nutmeg for the nervous** This elixir is ideal for people who think that they'll never conquer their fears. Sometimes they display the symptoms of genuine phobias: for example, fear of the dark, crowds or illness. Their fear is often accompanied by an extreme sensitivity to certain external circumstances: they might jump at the slightest noise or be unable to bear bright lights.

Nutmeg elixir, also known as mimulus, soothes fear and enables you to put things into their proper perspective. After a course of treatment, you feel better able to face life.

**Aspen for the anxious** This remedy is the answer for people who live in a state of perpetual paranoia and who can't stop imagining the worst in every situation. Sometimes, this condition can also be accompanied by nightmares and a persecution complex.

Aspen elixir helps you to come to terms with your sensitivity. You'll start to value it instead of regarding it with dread.

### ● ● ● DID YOU KNOW?

> If you're always worrying about other people and thus making your own life a misery, try red chestnut elixir. This will gradually reduce your need to put yourself in other people's shoes.

### KEY FACTS

* Take nutmeg elixir if you are constantly frightened, aspen elixir to quell thoughts of imminent catastrophe and red chestnut elixir to allow you to live your own life.

# 45 elixirs to boost morale

Some plant extracts can restore your joie de vivre. Fragile clematis and pungent mustard are the ones to try.

**Clematis: bringing dreamers back to reality** Edward Bach prescribed clematis elixir for the 'dozy ones', those who are never sufficiently awake to make a contribution in the world. They grow depressed, defeatist and sometimes even suicidal when forced to deal with reality. Clematis elixir enables them to become aware of what's going on around them and to join in. It also helps them find an outlet for dormant sensitivity and creativity. It is therefore an ideal means of restoring energy and morale.

**Mustard: escaping from the black hole** Mustard makes your palate tingle and stimulates your taste buds. Its elixir boosts the morale of the chronically melancholic, those people who feel as if they are permanently surrounded by a big, black cloud. A course of mustard elixir induces a feeling of optimism and reminds them that the sun always shines again after the rain.

### DID YOU KNOW?

> In addition to its oil and fruit, the olive tree is also the source of an elixir that helps those who've been finding life hard. It enables people who have been suffering psychologically and physically to regain their strength, vitality and enjoyment of life.

### KEY FACTS

* Clematis elixir helps melancholy dreamers to get back in touch with reality.

* Mustard elixir boosts the morale of depressed people close to despair.

* Olive elixir restores vitality to those who've been finding life difficult.

# 46
## try homeopathy

Homeopaths treat the body and mind together. Some of their remedies help drive away melancholy, correct defects of character and improve our relationship with the world. It would be a shame not to benefit from this type of treatment, especially as it has no harmful side-effects.

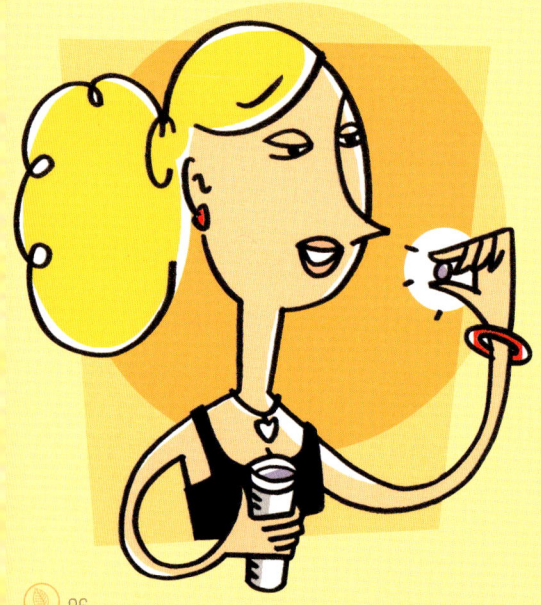

### More rigour and better treatments

When, at the end of the 18th century, Samuel Hahnemann established the foundations of homeopathy, Western medicine was still in its infancy. This German doctor was seeking a more rigorous approach on the part of doctors and more effective treatments. He stopped practising for several years in order to search for a more satisfactory method. Homeopathy is based on three principles: similarity (a substance can cure the very symptoms that it causes); minuscule amounts (the substance has to be administered in a greatly diluted form); individualized treatment (the patient, not a generalized illness, should be treated).

Homeopathic medicine still provokes controversy, but it is practised by many doctors in the medical establishment, as well as by homeopathic specialists.

## Curing moral faults

Some medicines are specifically intended to regulate moods. From the homeopathic point of view, emotional disorders are not distinct from the patient's physical condition and personal circumstances but are actually closely related to them, in exactly the same way physical symptoms are related. They can therefore be treated.

Anxiety, for example, can be treated with ignatia if it is caused by repeated annoyance; by aconite if it is completely irrational; and by arnica if it is the result of a recent severe emotional shock.

Other emotions and forms of behaviour that society tends to consider as moral flaws – such as jealousy, fear and a tendency to lie – can also be treated by homeopathic medicines.

### ● ● ● DID YOU KNOW?

> Homeopathic treatments for psychological problems need to be chosen after very thorough examination of the whole situation. It's difficult for us to choose the right medicine by ourselves, because we find it hard to judge our own circumstances accurately, so the choice of remedy is best left to a homeopathic doctor.

> There are often connections between certain physical symptoms and psychological aspects that help the doctor decide on the appropriate treatment. If chosen well, these remedies can bring rapid results.

### KEY FACTS

∗ Homeopathy can treat emotional disorders and also certain forms of behavioural dysfunction.

∗ In addition to anxiety, it can treat jealousy, fear, the tendency to lie and so on.

∗ The choice of remedy requires careful consideration and should be left to a homeopathic doctor.

# 47

## a bath fit for a goddess!

Are you envious of Cleopatra relaxing in her bath of asses' milk? Do you dream of pools surrounded by marble colonnades in Moorish palaces where you can lie amid rose-perfumed vapours and incense? You can treat yourself to a similar experience, even if it's on a slightly smaller scale.

### Nothing but relaxation

'I'm exhausted! I've had enough! Everyone's getting on my nerves! I just want to go home and lie in a lovely hot bath!' If that's how you feel when you're tense, anxious and annoyed, don't think twice: head straight for the bathroom.

A hot bath is a genuine anti-stress treatment, and it helps detox, too. The hot water dilates the blood vessels and the excretory organs work at full throttle.

### ●●● DID YOU KNOW?

> Perfume your bath with essential oils that make your skin shine like satin (neroli, rose, lavender).

> You can tailor your essential oils according to the time of day: relaxing oils in the evening (lavender, neroli) and invigorating ones in the morning (rosemary, cinnamon).

> Mix them in a spoonful of milk before pouring them under the bath taps so they spread evenly throughout the water.

Sitting in the water relaxes the inner ear, the organ responsible for keeping our balance when we stand. The steam clears the bronchial tubes, particularly if you put a few drops of essential oil into the bathwater. Finally, the heat relaxes the muscles and soothes the mind.

## Sound and light

You can make the experience even more memorable by creating the right setting. Light lots of coloured candles: don't use any other light source during your bath. Put on some relaxing music, but keep the volume low. Above all, make sure you won't be disturbed: unplug the telephone and don't answer the door if anyone rings the bell. The world can do without you for a while.

You'll feel completely relaxed after half an hour. Any more than that and you're liable to emerge pale and wrinkled! A good bath should not be too hot. The ideal time to take a bath is just before you go to bed: you'll emerge feeling so relaxed that you'll sleep like a baby.

If you take your bath during the day, make sure you have enough time for a rest afterwards. When you get out, wrap yourself in a warm dressing-gown and lie down for a quarter of an hour.

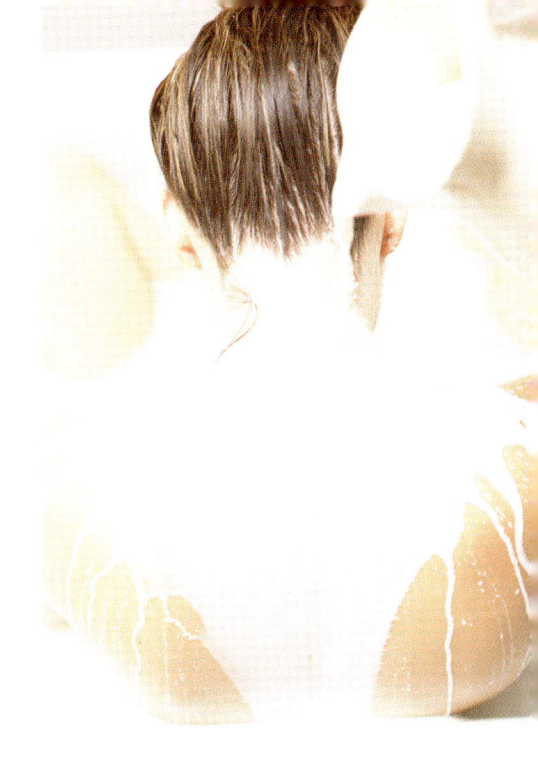

### KEY FACTS

* A hot bath is a genuine anti-stress and detox treatment.

* The heat dilates the blood vessels, the water soothes the muscles and the atmosphere calms the mind.

* Create the décor of your dreams with candles, music and fragrant oils.

# 48 let massage help you

If we experience stress for too long, we start to feel knots and tension in our muscles. The pain occurs in sensitive areas such as the upper and lower back, the neck and the shoulders.

## A sensation of well-being

Although we don't tend to think of it as such, the skin is a bodily organ with many functions. For example, it tells us about what is going on around us (heat, cold, rain, etc.) and makes us aware of any damage that has been done to us (burns, scratches). To perform these tasks, it is equipped with a multitude of sensory receptors linked to the nervous system. The information is then transmitted to the brain, where it is rapidly decoded so that we can react.

### ● ● ● DID YOU KNOW?

> Above all, massage makes us aware of the contours of our bodies. This may seem obvious, but we live in a society where touching is often still taboo outside of close relationships.

> We seldom have an opportunity to experience our bodies through the hands of another person outside of emotional and sexual relationships.

These same sensory receptors perceive the pleasant and soothing sensations of massage. But that's not all. A good massage relaxes muscles, loosens stiffened joints and stretches ligaments – it reaches the very places that are made painful by the accumulated stress.

## Specific forms of massage

Massage is therefore a good way of relieving physical tension and forgetting the worries that cause it. Some forms of massage have more specific purposes, such as the type of massage that concentrates on the meridians, or channels, along which our vital energy circulates (see Tip 37). As well as simply being relaxing, this form of massage also helps ensure the free flow of energy and generally improves the functioning of our bodily organs.

> However, this sensation plays an important part in the creation of self-image. We often have false images of ourselves, which cause negative attitudes and emotions.

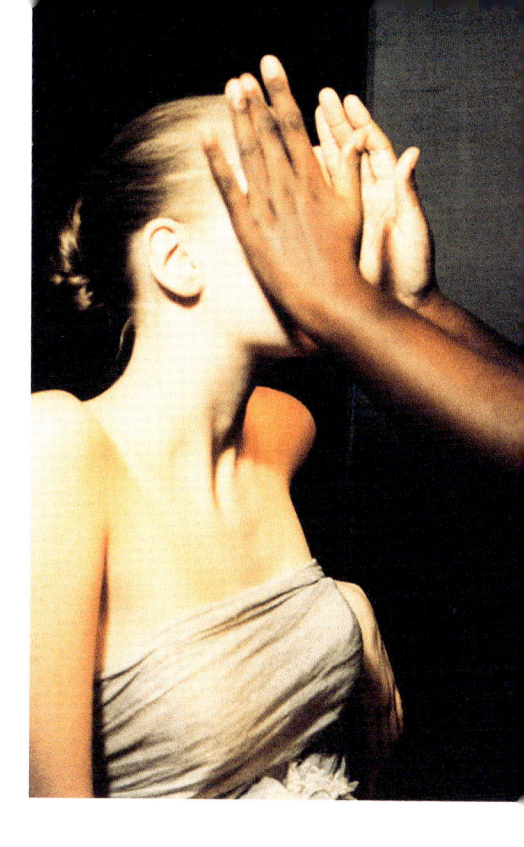

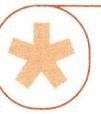

### KEY FACTS

* Our skin is a bodily organ equipped with a multitude of sensory receptors.

* Massage relieves tensions in the muscles and joints caused by stress.

## 49 upside-down breathing

Qi gong, a technique developed in traditional Chinese medicine, harmonizes the body's flow of vital energy. In China, it is practised by individuals in order to maintain good health but is also used as a treatment in specialist hospitals. It involves postures, sequences of gentle movement, breathing, etc.

**Tiredness, poor concentration and lack of alertness**

To drive away depression, relieve fatigue and remove stress, the Chinese suggest that we should breathe. That might not sound too challenging, but you can't do it just any old way. Among the host of exercises in Qi gong to harmonize energy flow is one that teaches us to breathe 'upside down'.

This inverted abdominal breathing is beneficial in many ways. It acts upon the meridians linked to the 'water' element: the kidneys and the bladder. Disruption to the

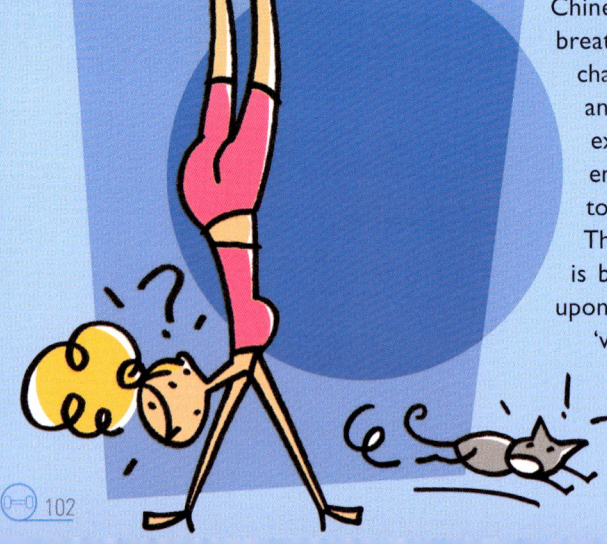

energy flow in these areas causes tiredness, lack of concentration, agitation, insomnia and loss of alertness.
To give yourself a boost during your detox programme and help combat all of these problems, try this special form of breathing.

## From bottom to top

The basic posture is the one used for meditation: sit cross-legged (on a cushion if this position hurts your knees), keeping your back and neck straight and pressing your chin slightly inwards. Close your eyes. Start to breathe in and simultaneously tense your perineum, the muscle that lies between the anus and the genital organs. Imagine a current rising from this area to the top of your head. Still breathing in, contract your abdominal muscles as if you want to lift your diaphragm up under your ribs. When the air reaches your lungs, let them swell and puff out your chest. Your lungs are now full of air. Breathe out by slowly relaxing first the chest, then the abdomen and finally the perineum.
Do this for several minutes every evening. It will gradually help you eliminate the tensions of the day and look forward positively to tomorrow.

### ●●● DID YOU KNOW?

> Energy to the kidneys, which is stimulated by this breathing exercise, is the most important kind in Chinese medicine. It is the fundamental energy that feeds all the others. It is also the sexual and reproductive energy. When its flow is seriously obstructed, the patient experiences fear, which might sometimes be intense and totally irrational.

### KEY FACTS

* Qi gong is a natural Chinese system of harmonizing the body's energy flow.

* Inverted abdominal breathing acts upon the energy of the kidneys and the bladder.

* It combats stress, tiredness and concentration problems.

# 50 close your eyes and visualize

If you complement the exercise in Tip 49 with a little visualization, it will make it even more effective. You simply need to relax and 'see' the energy circulating inside you.

**Heavenly energy flow!** To transform 'inverted abdominal breathing' into 'a little heavenly energy flow', Dr Yves Réquéna, acupuncturist and Qi gong specialist, suggests it should be accompanied by visualization. The exercise should be carried out in a relaxed state of mind. If necessary, practise a short relaxation session or do some deep breathing beforehand. You need to be relaxed to allow the images to form in your mind.

**Back and front** Now you're ready to begin. As you breathe in, concentrate your mind on the energy circulating within you and see it rising from your coccyx to the top of your head up your spine. As you breathe out, see it moving down the front of your body: from face to neck, chest and stomach.

### DID YOU KNOW?

> This visualization exercise was developed by ancient Taoist masters to improve the circulation of vital energy in the brain and spinal cord. The fundamental energy from the kidneys feeds these noble organs and enables them to function at their best.

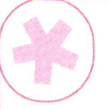

### KEY FACTS

* To make the inverted breathing exercise even more effective, try doing some visualization at the same time.

* Imagine the energy circulating inside you, climbing up the back of your body and descending down the front.

# 51 massage your solar plexus

There is another jin shin do (*do-in*) therapy that creates a feeling of calm. At the start of every day, massage the solar plexus to soothe away tension and anxiety.

**Some extraordinay channels!** According to Chinese medicine, the body contains an energy-distribution system. This meridian system consists of twelve main channels, each with specific, recognised acupuncture points. They carry energy to the organs, such as the kidney, heart and lungs, but there are eight extra-ordinary channels with various specific functions.

**The Ren Mai meridian** The points to stimulate in order to relieve anxiety and eliminate mental 'pollution' run along one of these extraordinary meridians, known as Ren Mai. It runs up the centre of the front of the body from the pubic region to just below the lower lip and contains a group of important pressure points in the region of the solar plexus. Massage this area vigorously, paying particular attention to the hollow just below the sternum.

### DID YOU KNOW?

> There are other stress-relieving points under and on the feet. They correspond to the beginning of the kidney meridian.
> One is in the hollow just below the tips of the toes. The other is in the lateral hollow of the arch.

### KEY FACTS

* In Jin shin do, points are massaged to relieve stress and anxiety.

* There are several important points that affect energy flow in the solar plexus.

* Other points are on and under the foot.

# 52
## don't skimp on magnesium

**To help your brain and nervous system to function, you need to feed them properly. Certain nutrients are absolutely vital to them if they are to control emotions and deal with excess tension.**

### A multitude of uses

Magnesium is a wonderful mineral that possesses myriad qualities: without it, the body would be unable to use vitamin C or the sugars it needs for fuel. Magnesium helps the body to utilize other minerals too, such as calcium, phosphorus and potassium. It metabolizes proteins and is necessary for muscle contraction, which is why we suffer from cramp when we don't have enough of it in our system.

### DID YOU KNOW?

> You might need magnesium supplements, particularly if you feel extremely nervous and mentally tired. They are available in several forms: capsules, tablets and drinkable phials.

> You can take up to 500mg per day without risk.

All that would be enough to rank it among the most vital minerals, but it has another, even more important function: it is essential for the transmission of impulses between nerve and brain cells. So, if you decide to make your detox programme as effective as possible by restoring order to your emotions and relieving nervous tension, make sure you consume enough magnesium. Otherwise, all your efforts may be in vain.

## Chocolate, hazelnuts and pulses

This needs to be stressed because often the body is starved of a decent supply of magnesium. There are two main reasons for the shortfall, both the result of modern Western lifestyles. Magnesium occurs in large quantities in dark chocolate, walnuts, hazelnuts, almonds and pulses (lentils, beans, chickpeas, etc.). In other words, it's in high-calorie foodstuffs that rarely make it on to slimming programmes. Cut out those types of food and you also cut out all the good sources of magnesium. While many miss out on magnesium because they are dieting, just as many rapidly exhaust the little they have because of stress. In times of stress, the body uses up much more magnesium than when it's in a state of calm. The simplest solution is to reintroduce the magnesium-rich foods mentioned above into your diet.

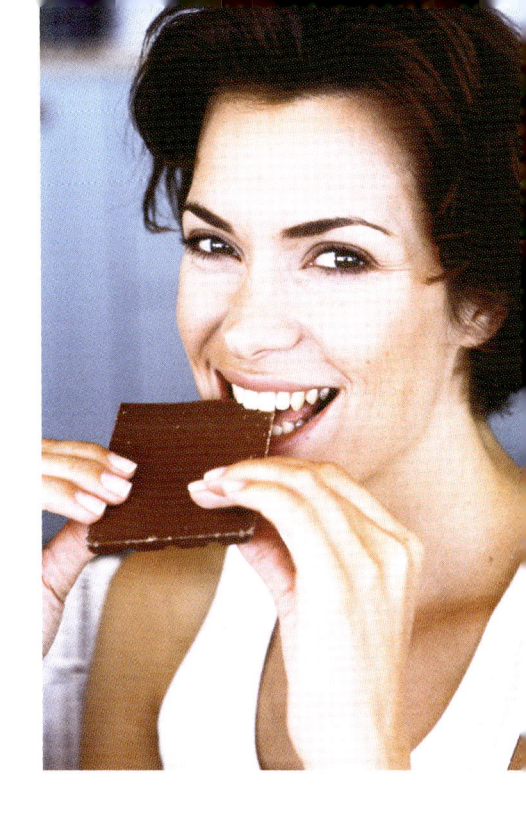

### KEY FACTS

* Magnesium is a vital mineral for the transmission of nerve impulses.

* To avoid a shortage of magnesium, eat chocolate, pulses and nuts or take magnesium supplements.

## 53 drive away negative thoughts

The 'pollution' in your head and heart can be cleansed. You just have to know how to do it. Learn how to cast out negative, painful and disturbing thoughts and replace them with happy ones.

### Always believing the worst

We are sometimes our own worst enemies by making our lives miserable. We can endlessly nurse bitter grievances just because of one annoying word or some unanswered request.

At other times, we insist on pessimistically fearing the worst instead of hoping for the best. In effect, we are manufacturing unnecessary worries and fears, although we may not consciously realize

### ●●● DID YOU KNOW?

> Positive visualization takes positive thinking a stage further by adding mental images to the process. You can do it with the help of a therapist or by yourself.

> A session begins with a brief period of relaxation exercises and then a scenario is developed that gives rise to positive sensations and emotions.

> Positive thinking undertaken under the guidance of a therapist would be followed by a discussion.

that we are doing this. We might dearly love to eliminate negative thoughts, but how do we go about it?

## As simple as saying, 'hello'

The answer is so simple that it beggars belief. Just make up your mind to do it. Each time a negative, pessimistic thought rears its ugly head, force yourself to reject it. At first, this may seem impossible, but by employing some will-power, you'll manage to get it out of your mind. It may only disappear for a few seconds, but that's a start! The more you practise, the better you'll be at keeping these destructive ideas at a distance.

You can also try positive thinking, a mental technique pioneered by the French pharmacist Emile Coué. At the beginning of the 20th century, he noticed that his medicines seemed to work better if he handed them over with a cheery word of encouragement. He did some further research on the subject, and eventually developed a system of mental programming that still inspires practitioners of positive thinking today. The method consists of formulating what you want to happen in short, simple, affirmative sentences, each containing a single idea. You then repeat them to yourself in a relaxed frame of mind.

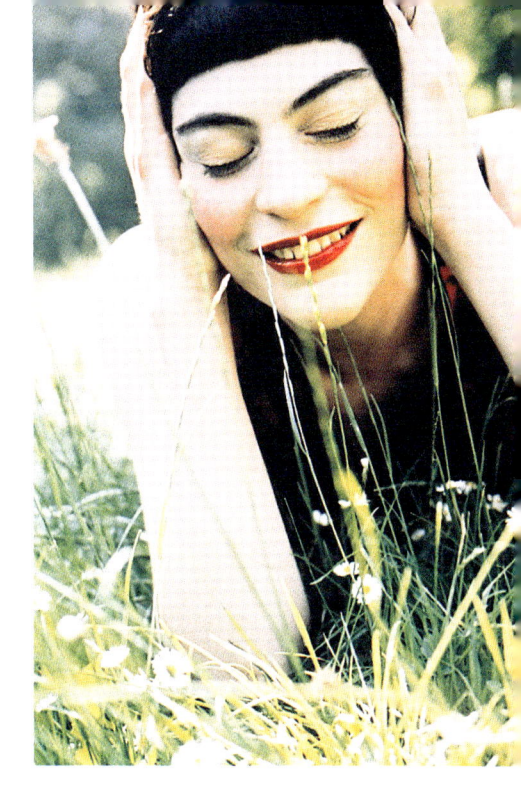

### KEY FACTS

* Don't endlessly dwell on dark and negative thoughts.

* Practise positive thinking. Add a visual and imaginary dimension to the process by trying positive visualization.

## 54 express yourself!

If you are discontent, you'll only make matters worse by suppressing your anger and keeping quiet about your unhappiness. You must learn how to express what you are feeling.

### A slow poison

Repressed, unexpressed emotions damage our minds, hearts and even our bodies. They cause frustration and resentment. They encourage destructive thoughts. Insidiously, they poison our relationships and ultimately disturb the way we function. Many physical ailments are the result of repressed emotions.

### ●●● DID YOU KNOW?

> If you are one of those people who can't rein in your emotions and find yourself hitting the roof over next to nothing, the same methods will work for you.

> They will enable you to distance yourself from the emotion that overwhelms you, allowing you to be in a better position to control it. You'll also escape the guilt that sneaks up on you afterwards.

Migraines, insomnia, high blood pressure and general aches and pains are sometimes just the body's roundabout way of dissipating excessive nervous tension. So, if you really want to cleanse yourself completely, you must learn to express your emotions.

## The fear of being judged

People who find it difficult to express what they feel are often worried about what others will think of them. They are worried about being judged and rejected. The first step towards changing this attitude is to acknowledge it and recognize its dangers.

Obviously, living in society means that there are certain aggressive impulses that we have to curb, but we shouldn't take this to extremes. Everyone has the right to self-expression, within limits. Assertiveness training offers a kind of education in self-expression. In the course of this education, the subject is faced with situations that demand a reaction. In each one, they make the effort to respond, succeed and gain confidence. Each successive situation is made more testing.

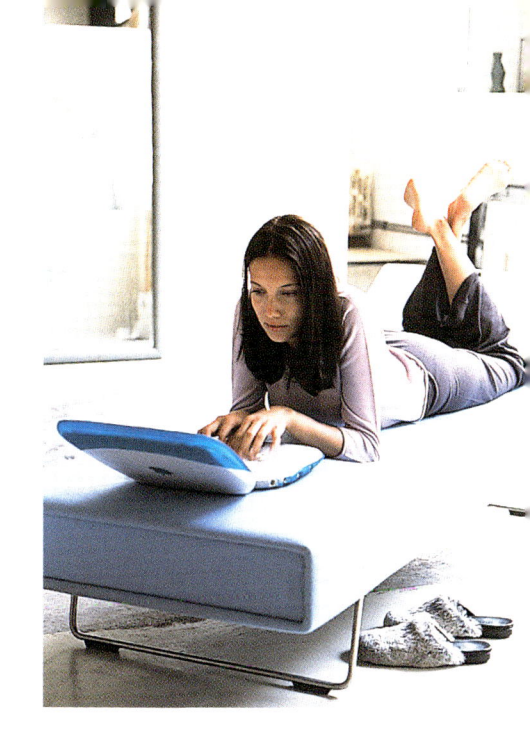

### KEY FACTS

* Unexpressed emotions can harm the mind, the heart and the body.

* Assertiveness training teaches you to express your emotions.

* These techniques are also helpful for those people who have trouble controlling their emotions.

# 55
## make them take 'no' for an answer

At one time or another, we have all felt obliged to agree to something we felt was wrong. Then we invent muddled reasons to justify our actions. We often do this because we are afraid to say no, or because we crave approval from the person making the request. We need to break the habit.

### It's about what we want

Some people agree to almost anything because they have a burning desire to be liked by everyone they meet. This is an extreme form of craving acceptance, but we all suffer from it from time to time, especially when confronted by someone who is persistent and confident that they are in the right. The temptation will always be there to go along with their suggestions.

### ● ● ● DID YOU KNOW?

> To learn to say 'no', we must first be aware of some false ideas we have about ourselves.

> You don't become popular by just agreeing to everything someone asks. Sometimes this merely encourages others to use you.

However, if we agree against our better judgement, the contradiction causes an inner conflict. At first, this might remain hidden, but eventually the tension will come out in one form or another, such as tiredness, depression or irritability. We can't constantly suppress our own wishes in favour of those of others.

## The 'no' phase

The inability to say 'no' starts in childhood. At around two years, all children go through a 'no' phase. They take delight in repeating the word all day long, rejecting everything suggested to them. By doing so, they gain their first experience of independence from their mother and family. But this is also a very frustrating time for children, who are unable to articulate what they want or need. If they are met with parental anger, it might be many years before they are able to assert themselves again.

Constantly suppressing your wishes and feelings might 'pollute' you with myriad mental and emotional problems. However, with patience and determination, you can learn how to say 'no' again.

> By saying 'no' to someone you are refusing one specific request, not rejecting that person as a whole. Asserting that you are an individual with your own wishes is a way of showing respect and affection for other people.

### KEY FACTS

∗ Agreeing to everything causes nervous tension that eventually results in illness.

∗ Self-assertion is learnt in childhood but it's never too late to get back into the habit of standing up for yourself.

# 56
## stop feeling guilty

**A sense of a guilt is the worst form of mental poison. It can be exploited by others to achieve their own ends. If it's not banished, it forms a prison for our minds.**

### A misguided feeling

Don't confuse true guilt with a sense of guilt. The first indicates that you have done something wrong, but nobody is infallible. If we are honest with ourselves and other people, we should be able to acknowledge our errors, to ask for forgiveness and, in most cases, find a resolution.

A sense of guilt is very different. This phrase refers to that vague, subjective

### ●●● DID YOU KNOW?

> To free yourself of a sense of guilt, you must first learn to stop deceiving yourself.
> Then, love the child you were, including all that you experienced, and forgive your own errors.

> Nobody is completely innocent, nor completely guilty: use that as your starting point to rebuilding your self-confidence.

feeling that there must always be a reason why we should reproach ourselves. It means we are always ready to accept responsibility for whatever goes wrong, whether it's our fault or not. We won't allow ourselves to succeed as we don't want to outperform other people. We won't let ourselves love or be loved because we believe we don't deserve it. This capacity to feel guilty for each and every thing is like going through life wearing a ball and chain.

## Why are you always so stupid?

A serious guilt complex requires a course of psychotherapy, perhaps a long one. However, this is unnecessary for most people, who simply need to lose a habit that developed during childhood. A child who witnesses a sad event, such as the death of a grandparent or the departure of a sibling, without having it explained to them will automatically place the blame for it squarely on their own shoulders. If, in addition, the child is bombarded with thoughtless comments such as 'Why are you always so stupid?', they will be unable to overcome the sense of guilt.

If you suffer from this, you must work back to the time when you picked up this destructive habit, then gradually rebuild your self-confidence.

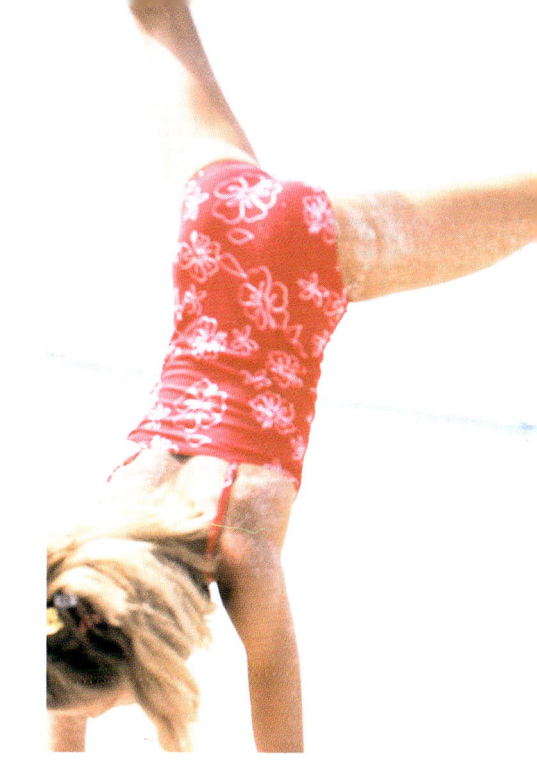

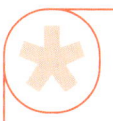

### KEY FACTS

* We must not confuse genuine guilt with a sense of guilt.

* Having a sense of guilt means feeling guilty without cause or justification.

* To eradicate it, we must gradually rebuild our self-confidence.

# 57 drive out the green-eyed monster

**Jealousy is an emotion that poisons our whole existence. It gradually wears us down, damaging our relationships and gnawing away at our peace of mind. Sometimes it can dominate our lives. If you want peace of mind, drive out jealousy.**

## Masochistic martyrdom

Jealousy does, to some extent, have a positive psychological role to play. It drives us to defend our territory and define its limits more clearly. It acts like a psychological fuel to provide us with the energy and aggression to act and react. However, it often spirals out of control. When this happens, it dominates us, obscures the truth and makes us irrational. We become the victim of a slow,

### ● ● ● DID YOU KNOW?

> Here are some ideas for dealing with jealousy as soon as it rears its ugly head.
> When you feel suspicion beginning to grow, consider immediately whether you are asking yourself the right questions.

> Jealousy is not a failing; nor is it an immutable part of your character that you cannot address. It's neurotic behaviour that can be overcome.
> Jealousy is more painful than any real betrayal. Realizing this will help cure you of it.

silent torture, an entirely masochistic martyrdom. Suspicion soon becomes as natural as breathing.

The principal problem with jealousy is that it has no connection with reality. We spend our time reacting to our imaginations and fantasies. But, although they are all in our mind, they never give us a moment's peace.

## Jealousy can be found anywhere

The most familiar breeding ground for jealousy is in a couple relationship, but it can also develop among friends, neighbours and parents and children. The only thing really needed is for one person to suspect the other of some unpardonable betrayal.

Pathological jealousy, of course, needs to be treated by a psychotherapist. As with so many problems, its root can be traced back to early childhood. However, the little bouts of jealousy that everyone experiences at one time or another can be cured if we take a step back from our fantasies and try to look at them rationally. It's certainly worth making this effort, because there's nothing like the sense of freedom and the peace of mind you experience when the poisonous monster has been driven out. Your whole life will be better for it.

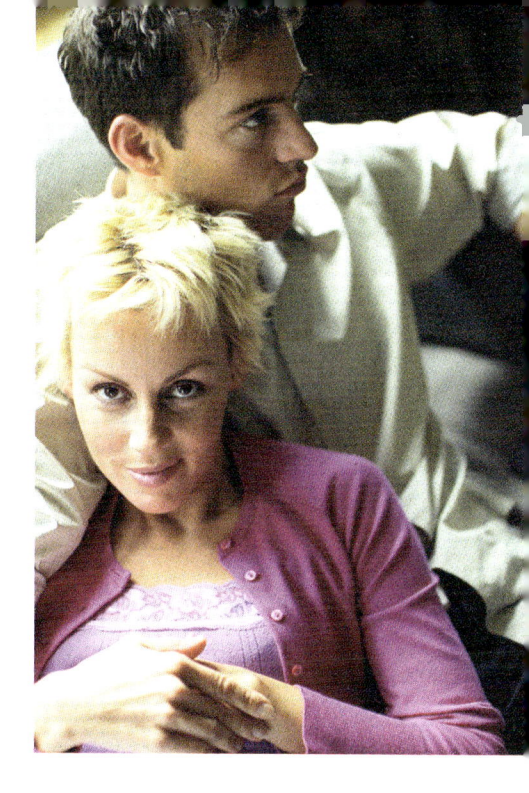

### KEY FACTS

* Jealousy afflicts us like a kind of poison.

* It has nothing to do with reality but feeds on imagination and fantasy.

* To cure ourselves of it, we need to distance ourselves from our fantasies.

# 58 make a date with nature

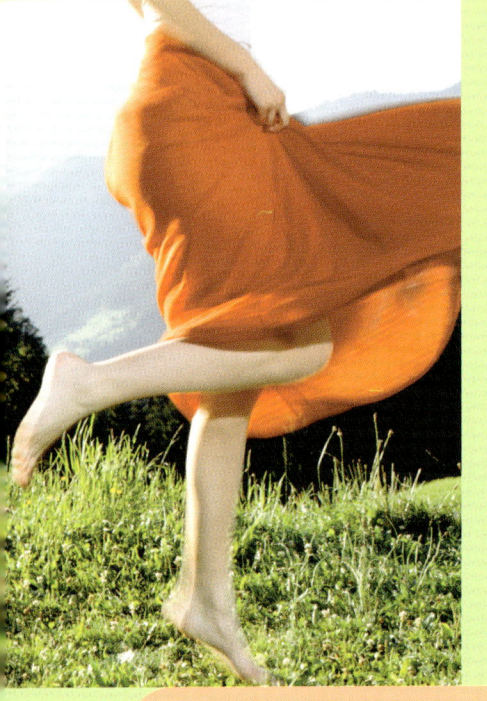

So you are detoxed, purified inside and out. You have cleansed your body of its toxins, your mind of its negativity. Your relationships are less complicated and your emotions are under control. To help preserve this contented state of mind and body, go for a regular walk in the woods.

### DID YOU KNOW?

> Ions are electric particles found in the air. Some are charged positively, others negatively.

> They are created by the interaction of solar rays, photosynthesis in trees and water spray (waves, waterfalls and so on). There are fewer negative ions and they are more fragile than positive ions.

## A healthy boost

Nature provides us with everything we need to pursue a perfect detox programme: for instance, food, medicinal herbs, clay and pure air. But even when you're not in the midst of a programme, it can still give you a healthy boost. A simple walk in the woods, for example, is enough to make you feel as good as new. There you will inhale air that is healthier, purer and richer in negative ions. You will be taking gentle exercise, which will help the oxygen reach the extremities of your body and accelerate your blood circulation. You will breathe in the essences of trees that will clean your lungs or calm your anxiety. Finally, you will give your ears respite from the noise of modern life and treat them to the sounds of birdsong, the chirruping of insects and the rustle of leaves as the wind blows through the trees.

## Take a little time out

Try to enjoy a country walk at least twice a month. Go by yourself or with someone who shares your attitude to the countryside. Avoid chatterboxes who will spoil the peace and quiet. Keep well away from anyone liable to disturb the atmosphere. Choose a secluded spot that other walkers are not likely to visit and take a little time out. Sit at the foot of a tree, close your eyes and let your thoughts wander where they will. Gradually they will fade and you will feel at peace with the world.

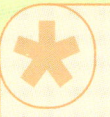

### KEY FACTS

* A walk in the woods is a detox treatment in its own right.

* It gives you physical exercise, negative ions and a sense of peace.

* Make sure you choose a quiet spot and the right person to accompany you, then just relax at the foot of a tree.

> They are, however, very good for us. They are rapidly destroyed in an enclosed room but in open countryside we inhale them and give ourselves a healthy boost.

# 59 take a seaside holiday

**If you prefer the seaside to the woods, save up and treat yourself to a course of thalassotherapy. Take advantage of all the sea's many health-giving resources.**

### Hot or cold sea water

The sea is extraordinarily rich in therapeutic resources, particularly minerals. A litre of sea water contains millions of mineral particles. Fortunately, we don't have to drink it to reap the benefits. All we need to do is jump in the sea and these marvellous substances will be absorbed through the skin.

That's basically how thalassotherapy works. Various treatments involving hot

● ● ● DID YOU KNOW?

> You can drink sea water, if you really want to. It's available in drinkable phials and is a good treatment for tiredness and overindulgence, as its composition is very similar to that of human blood serum.

> Courses of these phials last two or three weeks, and it's best to take them at the start of a new season.

or cold sea water are available, such as baths, whirlpools, jet showers and gentler affusion showers. Apart from the immediate pleasure they provide, these treatments regenerate the body and rid it of toxins. A good course of thalassotherapy is the ideal starting point for a detox programme. Sea water is a very effective cleanser, as it stimulates the excretory organs and expels toxins.

## Starting as you mean to go on

There are many thalassotherapy resorts throughout the world. Some are famous for the treatment of specific complaints, such as insomnia, arthritis or helping people quit smoking, but all offer basic treatments that are excellent ways to combat stress and fatigue, and to cleanse the body.

During a course of thalassotherapy, which lasts a week, you usually have four treatments each day. These are chosen at the beginning of your stay in consultation with the doctor at the centre, who will tailor the programme to your particular needs (and sometimes your preferences). All the resorts offer health-food menus, and a dietician is on hand to give advice, sometimes even lessons on healthy cooking. All in all, it's a fine way to embark on a healthy new lifestyle.

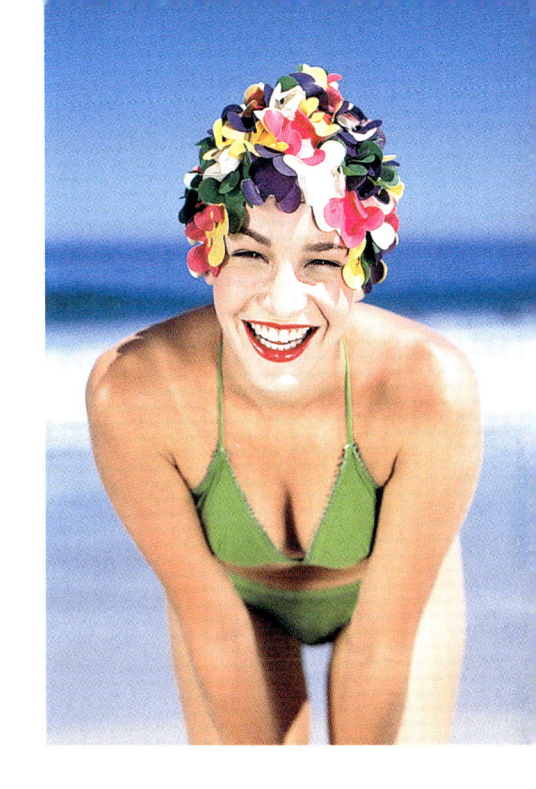

### KEY FACTS

* Thalassotherapy involves treatments using sea water.

* Sea water is rich in minerals to recharge and cleanse the body.

* The treatments take place under medical supervision and often with the guidance of a dietician.

# 60 enjoy it!

A detox programme is not a punishment. It will be most effective if you actually enjoy it. You are not doing it to deprive yourself but to discover the pleasure of a healthy lifestyle.

**Get in touch with your inner being** Some people finish a detox programme feeling light and exhilarated, while others are despondent as they've had to deprive themselves of so much. If you haven't enjoyed the detox, you'll find it hard to keep up your new good habits when the programme is over.

**Anything's good if it works** Detoxing is not always wholly pleasant. You will eat some things that taste bad (at least at first) and deprive yourself of foods that you love. But you can add moments of pure pleasure to your programme to help you over the rough patches. Make some time for yourself. Have a light snack while watching a favourite film. Read that long novel you always promised yourself. Treat your skin to some natural beauty masks. Enjoy the experience in any way that you can.

### DID YOU KNOW?

> To ensure your detox programme is a happy experience, you need to choose the right time to do it.
> Don't embark on a detox programme at a time when you've got too many worries and commitments. You will find it far too hard to commit yourself.

### KEY FACTS

* A detox programme will always be more successful if you enjoy it.

* Build in some little treats every now and again and spare some time for yourself.

# case study

**Now my relationships are better for me**

«The first time I followed a mono-diet, it was by accident. I was feeling heavy, unattractive and down in the dumps, so I followed what I thought was a slimming diet in a magazine. I found out later it was actually a detox programme. It was badly explained and not aimed at the right audience, but it certainly worked. At the end of a week I felt much lighter, so I found out more about this treatment. I read up on it and consulted a specialist in natural medicine, who has been treating me now for some years. Gradually, with the detox programmes I've been doing every three months (usually at the start of each new season), I've learnt how to make my behaviour, my emotions and, above all, my relationships 'less polluted' and better for me. I've come to understand why and how I used to let myself be used by people. Many aspects of my life have become clearer. I've put an end to relationships that were bad for me and I've finally dared to make friends with like-minded people. It's taken a lot of hard work and it's not over yet, but I know I'm on the right path.»

# useful addresses

## » Acupuncture

**British Acupuncture Council**
63 Jeddo Road
London W12 9HQ
tel: 020 8735 0400
www.acupuncture.org.uk

**British Medical
Acupuncture Society**
12 Marbury House
Higher Whitley, Warrington
Cheshire WA4 4QW.
tel: 01925 730727

**Australian Acupuncture
and Chinese Medicine
Association**
PO Box 5142
West End, Queensland 4101
Australia
www.acupuncture.org.au

## » Herbal medicine

**British Herbal Medicine
Association**
Sun House, Church Street
Stroud, Gloucester GL5 1JL
tel: 01453 751389

**National Institute
of Medical Herbalists**
56 Longbrook Street
Exeter, Devon EX4 6AH
tel: 01392 426022

## » Homeopathy

**British Homeopathic
Association**
Hahnemann House
29 Park Street West
Luton LU1 3BE
tel: 0870 444 3950

**The Society of Homeopaths**
4a Artizan Road
Northampton NN1 4HU
tel: 01604 621400

**Australian Homeopathic
Association**
PO Box 430, Hastings
Victoria 3915, Australia
www.homeopathyoz.org

## » Massage

**British Massage Therapy
Council**
www.bmtc.co.uk

**Association of British
Massage Therapists**
42 Catharine Street
Cambridge CB1 3AW
tel: 01223 240 815

**European Institute of Massage**
42 Moreton Street
London SW1V 2PB
tel: 020 7931 9862

## » Qi Gong

**Qi Gong Association
of America**
PO Box 252
Lakeland, MN, USA
email: info@nqa.org

**World Natural Medicine
Foundation**
College of Medical Qi Gong
9904 106 Street,
Edmonton AB T5K 1C4
Canada

## » Relaxation therapy

**British Autogenic Society**
The Royal London
Homoeopathic Hospital
Greenwell Street
London W1W 5BP

**British Complementary
Medicine Association**
PO Box 5122
Bournemouth BH8 0WG
tel: 0845 345 5977

## » Yoga

**The British Wheel of Yoga**
25 Jermyn Street
Sleaford, Lincs NG34 7RU
tel: 01529 306 851
www.bwy.org.uk

# index

| | | | | | | |
|---|---|---|---|---|---|---|
| **A**cne | 56 | Hot-water bottle | 66 | **R**aw food | 26 |
| Alcohol | 22 | | | Reflexology | 60 |
| Animal proteins | 24 | **I**nhalation | 80 | Relaxation | 88, 90 |
| Anxiety | 90 | Intestines | 74, 76, 78 | | |
| Aromatic herbs | 18 | | | **S**auna | 50 |
| Assertiveness training | 110 | **J**ealousy | 116 | Sea water | 120 |
| | | Jin shin do | 78, 106 | Self-assertion | 112 |
| **B**aths | 98 | | | Skin | 56, 100 |
| Bowel movements | 38 | **K**idneys | 36, 44, 62 | Slimming | 46 |
| Breathing | 80, 82, 102 | | | Smoking | 20 |
| | | **L**aughter | 77 | Sophrology | 90 |
| **C**hocolate | 106 | Liver | 30, 34, 66, 70, 78, 85 | Stomach | 78 |
| Clay | 41, 64, 65 | | | Stress | 88 |
| Cleansing | 18 | Lungs | 80 | Sweating | 50, 52 |
| Charcoal | 66 | Lymphatic drainage | 58 | | |
| Colonic irrigation | 76 | | | **T**ea | 44 |
| Constipation | 72 | **M**agnesium | 106 | Thalassotherapy | 120 |
| Cooking | 26 | Massage | 60, 78, 100 | | |
| | | Meat | 24 | **V**egetable oils | 16 |
| **E**ssential oils | 98 | Monodiets | 31 | Vegetables | 34, 36 38 |
| Exercise | 52, 72, 88 | | | Visualization | 104 |
| | | **N**ature | 118 | | |
| **D**o-in | 78, 106 | Nuts | 106 | **W**ater | 12, 72 |
| | | | | Weight | 20, 46, 47 |
| **F**asting | 32 | **O**live oil | 68 | Wine | 22 |
| Feet | 60 | Olive tree | 68 | | |
| Fibre | 42, 72 | Organic food | 14 | | |
| Fish | 24 | | | | |
| Floral elixirs | 92 | **P**lants | 54, 56, 62, 70, 74, 82, 83 | | |
| Fruit | 28, 30, 31, 34, 36, 38, 40 | Pleasure | 122 | | |
| | | Positive thinking | 108 | | |
| **G**uilt (sense of) | 114 | Poultices | 64 | | |
| | | Pulses | 106 | | |
| **H**erbal teas | 54, 62, 68 | | | | |
| Herbs | 18 | **Q**i gong | 102 | | |
| Homeopathy | 96 | | | | |

125

# acknowledgements

Cover: Kactus/Photonica; p. 8-9: Pinto/Zefa; p.11: V. Besnault/Getty Images; p.13: R. and M. Deren/Marie Claire; p.15: Cole/Zefa; p.17: Emely/Zefa; p.19: A. Peisl/Zefa; p.21: R. Knobloch/Zefa; p. 23: J. Dunn/Photonica; p. 24: C. Gullung/Photonica; p. 26-27: Neo Vision/Photonica; p. 29: R. Seagraves/Photonica; p. 32: Gerd George/Getty Images; p.35: Cole/Zefa; p. 37: Neo Vision/Photonica; p. 39: S. Lancrenon/Marie Claire; p. 43: A. Green/Zefa; p. 44: Emely/Zefa; p. 48-49: T. Nogushi/Photonica; p. 51: Möllenberg/Zefa; p. 53: H. Winkler/Zefa; p. 54-55: Neo Vision/Photonica; p. 56: Auslöser/Zefa; p. 59: D. Jaffe/Getty Images; p. 61: A. Beer/Marie France; p. 62: T. Allofs/Zefa; p. 65: W. Maldonado/Getty Images; p. 69: B. Sporrer/Zefa; p. 70-71: Neo Vision/Photonica; p. 72: M. Thomsen/Zefa; p.75: VCL George/Getty Images; p.81: H. Winkler/Zefa; p.82: G. de Chabaneix/Marie Claire; p.86-8: P. Scholey/Getty Images; p. 89: BP/E. Buis/Zefa; p. 90-91: A. Neunsinger/Getty Images; p.92: Creasource/Zefa; p.99: H. Noleman/Photonica; p.101: L. Deren/Marie Claire; p.107: J. Darell/Getty Images; p.109: Emely/Zefa; p.111: Cora/Marie Claire; p.112-113: E. Bernager/Zefa; p.115: A. Peisl/Zefa; p.117: Gerd George/Getty Images; p.118: K. Solveig/Zefa; p.121: Pinto/Zefa.

Illustrations: Philippe Doro pages 78, 96 and 102.

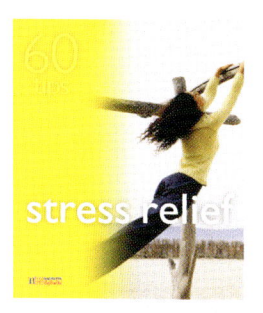

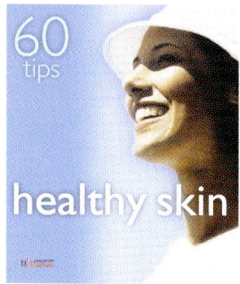

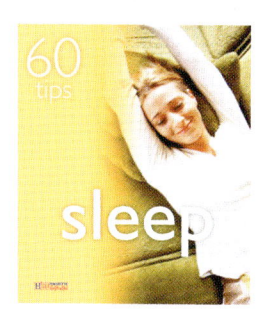

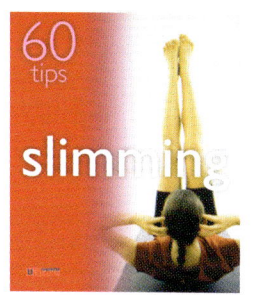

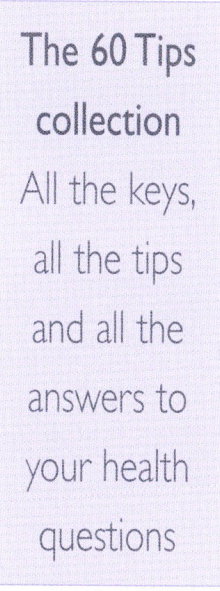

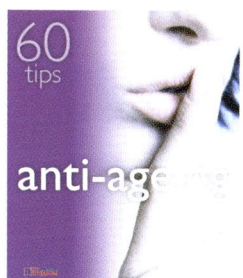

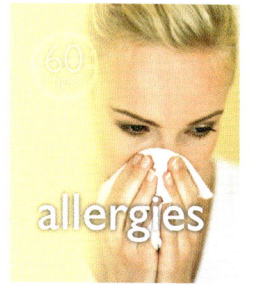

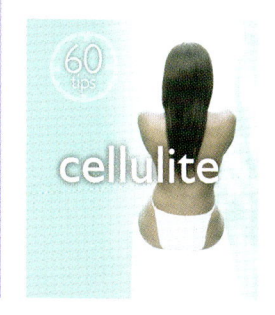

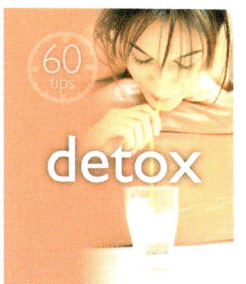

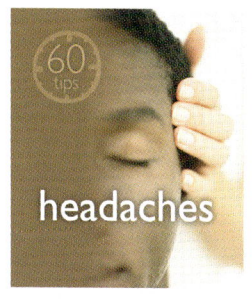

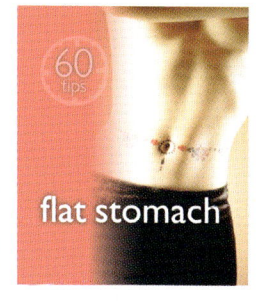

| 60 tips stress relief | 60 tips healthy skin | 60 tips sleep |
| --- | --- | --- |
| 60 tips slimming | **The 60 Tips collection** — All the keys, all the tips and all the answers to your health questions | 60 tips anti-ageing |
| 60 tips allergies | | 60 tips cellulite |
| 60 tips detox | 60 tips headaches | 60 tips flat stomach |

Series editor: Marie Borrel

Editorial directors: Caroline Rolland and Delphine Kopff

Editorial assistants: Delphine Kopff and Anne Vallet

Graphic design and layout: G & C MOI

Final checking: Chloé Chauveau and Fanny Morel

Illustrations: Guylaine Moi

Production: Felicity O'Connor

Translation: JMS Books LLP

© Hachette Livre (Hachette Pratique) 2003
This edition published in 2005 by Hachette Illustrated UK, Octopus Publishing Group Ltd.,
2–4 Heron Quays, London E14 4JP

English translation by JMS Books LLP (email: moseleystrachan@blueyonder.co.uk)
Translation © Octopus Publishing Group Ltd.

All rights reserved. No part of this publication may be reproduced in material form (including photocopying or storing it in any medium by electronic means and whether or not transiently or incidentally to some other use of this publication) without the written permission of the copyright owner, except in accordance with the provisions of the Copyright, Designs and Patents Act 1988 or under the terms of a licence issued by the Copyright Licensing Agency, 90 Tottenham Court Road, London W1P 9HE.

A CIP catalogue for this book is available from the British Library

ISBN-13: 978-1-84430-092-1

ISBN-10: 1-84430-092-7

Printed in Singapore by Tien Wah Press